50 Ways
to a
Healthy
Heart

If you wish to be more informed about health matters, please contact Professor Christiaan Barnard directly at:

www.askbarnard.com
– a service of the Christiaan Barnard Foundation.

50 Ways to a Healthy Heart

Professor Christiaan Barnard

Thorsons

Thorsons
An Imprint of HarperCollins*Publishers*
77–85 Fulham Palace Road,
Hammersmith, London W6 8JB

The Thorsons website address is: www.thorsons.com

Published by Thorsons 2001

10 9 8 7 6 5 4 3 2

A catalogue record for this book
is available from the British Library

ISBN 0 00 712224 1

Printed and bound in Great Britain by
Martins the Printers Ltd, Berwick upon Tweed

Contents

Introduction

For me the heart has always been an organ without any mystique attached to it. It is of relatively simple construction; it only has one function, and more research has gone into it and its workings than into almost anything else in our bodies. And yet – no other organ is respected more than the heart; neither the lungs nor the kidneys nor the liver, although these organs are much more complicated than the heart. Even today we do not know everything about the workings of the liver, for instance.

The heart is merely a primitive pump. It basically consists of four parts: muscles, nerves, arteries, and valves. This wondrous organ has only one task to perform in our bodies – it pumps blood.

I have often thought about it when I was doing a heart transplant: by removing the heart from the donor we deprive that organ of its only function. For an hour or more the donor-heart could truly be said to lie before our very eyes – embedded in ice. There was nothing mysterious about it anymore. The heart had lost its magic.

I could never quite understand why historical and literary references to this organ go so far back in recorded history. I once took the time to go through the Bible. It seems incredible, but it contains more than 300 references to the heart. The liver, meanwhile, is only mentioned once.

One need only think of literature and music. How many quotations, how many idioms are there in which the word 'heart' plays a central role? From classical literature to romance novels, from opera to modern pop music – the heart is omnipresent.

> *I have never heard anyone singing: "My kidney is in the highlands."*

In his wonderful book *The Mythology of the Heart*, the Swiss internist Dr. Frank Nager gives an impressive description of the importance of this organ in the thinking of all cultures. The heart was a symbol. It has been thought to be the center of life, the source of our intellect, our will, our courage, our feelings, and our emotions. It should be the source of religiousness and wisdom, the fertile soil of the soul. According to Erich Fried, the language of symbols is the only language which everyone should learn.

Five thousand years ago the Sumerians of Babylon praised the heart in their poetry as the center of all emotions. This attitude towards the heart has also been found in the ancient cultures of the Greeks, the Chinese, and the Aztecs. When the ancient Egyptians mummified their dead, they removed all internal organs – except the heart. It was unthinkable for them that there could be a life after death without the most important source of life: the heart. For the Egyptians a "heartless person" was not someone who showed little feeling; they simply thought of such a person as a fool.

> *In some cultures the heart was taken out of the body after death and weighed. But the heaviest heart was not considered the best; it was always the lightest heart that was most highly esteemed. This may be the reason why we still maintain today that one should learn to live "light-heartedly."*

Matisse, Munch, Murillo, Shakespeare, Hölderlin, and Goethe – all great artists – very frequently put the heart in the center of their most important work. With Matisse it was a small red dot in his painting *Icarus*; Munch portrayed the right hand over the left side of the chest in his masterpiece *The Separation*; with Murillo the heart of a young man even bursts into flames after being pierced by an arrow. There are countless examples of the importance of the heart in visual art.

Quite frankly, I find this rather overdone.

However, I would also find it somewhat strange to say to a woman "I love you with all my liver" or "I love you with all my spleen." It sounds much better if we say "with all my heart," but are we not overrating the heart here?

I think I know why we do this. We do not experience any other organ, any other part of our body, as immediately as the heart. It is the only organ in our body that reacts directly to stress and emotional events. If we are frightened, angry, stressed, or even when we fall in love, our heart is the first organ to react to this. It beats louder, faster, sending out signals. You do not listen to your liver or to your kidneys when these are excited. You only feel your heart. This does rather justify what was said about the heart in earlier cultures: that it houses our emotions.

As I understand the Bible, God initially did not put much value on the heart when He created man. It is surprising, but in Genesis it is written that God's most important act of creation was to breathe life into man. It is interesting to note that in many languages the word for breath and the word for soul are the same or similar. I wish Aristotle had read Genesis, because he was convinced that the heart was the seed of the soul.

> *The "secret" of our heart: it is the only organ that we can feel in times of great excitement.*

Even in the thousands of years that have passed, the mystique attached to the heart has not been lost – a fact that many charlatans have used to their advantage.

I would like to illustrate this with a little story about a man who was a friend of mine as well as being world famous. For many years I had a very close friendship with the comedian, writer, and film star Peter Sellers. One day he came to Cape Town with Lynn Frederick, his wife at the time, to take part in a backgammon match. During this time we also spent several pleasant hours together, and my wife and I arranged to meet up with them again a few weeks later in Rome. When we met up, Peter chartered a yacht in Ostia near Rome and the four of us went off to sea. As we neared the end of our cruise he came to me and showed me an EKG. He asked me for my medical opinion without telling me whose EKG it was. I could see at a glance that the owner of that EKG needed to see a doctor at once.

"It's *my* EKG," Peter admitted. I immediately offered to organize the best cardiologist and a hospital bed in Cape Town for him. He agreed. As I had to attend a conference overseas, my wife Barbara was to look after him for the first few days. She spent a long time waiting for him at Cape Town's airport, but he never came although his name actually appeared on the passenger list. We heard nothing from him after that.

About three months later I was invited to a birthday party given by King Hussein of Jordan. And whom did I meet to my great surprise and joy among the many guests? Peter Sellers. He appeared relieved to see me, and he told me straightaway what had happened. Upon hearing my offer that he be examined in Cape Town, he had immediately chartered a plane and departed – but not for South Africa. He flew to southeast Asia, to Manila in the Philippines – to the notorious spiritual healers there.

Allow me a short personal observation at this point. Basically I am one of those doctors who believe that nothing between heaven and earth is absolutely impossible. I would be the last to deny the truth and seriousness of phenomena we cannot scientifically explain. But I am also the first to point a finger at those who would take advantage of others, at those who exploit the fears of people worried about their health.

In the case of Peter Sellers it was perfectly clear to me: whatever he should choose to do afterwards, Western medicine would first have to deal with his heart condition. His EKG had shown quite clearly that he only had a short time to live.

At that party given by King Hussein, Peter Sellers, who had a very poor opinion of Western medicine and a very high one of mystics, said to me: "Congratulate me, Chris, I have been healed; I am perfectly healthy again. Eleven operations were necessary and the faith healers operated with their bare hands. [One] ... opened my chest with his finger and at the first operation he took out the blood clot and showed it to me [this was more likely probably a chicken liver]. There was blood everywhere. At the end I decided to have my appendix out as well. I have no scar but [the] appendix had been removed. I feel born again."

I only nodded my head, not knowing what to say at first. A very happy man who considered himself fully recovered stood before me. I, on the other hand, knew about the charlatans in the Philippines, who are very deft at removing "diseased tissue" from the body.

When I found my voice again I said to Peter, "Do me a favor, please go to a cardiologist and have yourself examined. If he confirms what you are telling me, I swear to you I will publicly admit that we of the medical profession are not really necessary for the treatment of illnesses anymore."

I never saw the great comedian Peter Sellers again. Two months later he was dead. The cause of death: a heart attack.

> *"I have been healed," Peter Sellers told me after his visit to the faith healers. Shortly after that he was dead.*

Today I believe that so many people do not have to die of a heart attack. The heart is a very well-researched organ. We know about most of the risk factors that can lead to a heart attack. We know how we should live and what is bad for us. If you have healthy eating habits, lead an active life and guide your stress into the right channels, you will significantly reduce the risk of a heart attack. Nevertheless, cardiovascular diseases remain the number one cause of death in all industrialized countries. More than half of all deaths result from a heart condition, and the numbers are still rising.

This is the reason I am writing this book. I was a surgeon for decades. I could help many whose heart was already irreparably damaged. But I believe that in the vast majority of cases it need not get this far. Heart conditions are seldom inherent; we "acquire" them in the course of our lives because we do not treat our body as well as it deserves. We know today that only 20% of those diagnosed with a heart condition are found to be more at risk for genetic reasons. In all other cases, lifestyle has practically predetermined their eventual condition.

> *Men are more likely to have a heart attack, older women who have a heart attack are more likely to die from it.*

The American Heart Association has listed the most important risk factors of cardiovascular diseases:

- Age
  Four out of five people who die of a heart attack are older than 65. Women who have an attack at this age die of it twice as often as men.
- Sex
  Men are more likely to have a heart attack, and their attacks hit them earlier in life than women.
- Descent
  There is no doubt that certain heart conditions are hereditary. If there is a family history of a heart condition, you are more likely to get one yourself.
- Smoking
  Smokers have heart attacks twice as often as non-smokers. We know today that passive smokers also run more risk of heart disease.
- High blood pressure
  High blood pressure forces the heart to work harder. It causes enlargement of the heart and changes in the arteries, causing the heart to weaken.
- High cholesterol level
  I will explain the latest findings in this regard in Chapter 9.
- Too little exercise
  This is a risk factor of increasing importance. Thirty minutes of sport three times a week is sufficient.
- Overweight
  If you are carrying too many pounds around with you, you are overtaxing your heart. Being overweight also has a negative influence on blood pressure and blood fat levels.
- Diabetes mellitus
  More than 80% of people with diabetes die of a heart problem. Such people have to take special care of their bodies.

- Stress
  Stress itself is less often the cause of a heart attack, but its "concomitant circumstances" such as smoking, eating the wrong foods, and lack of exercise are usually to blame.

I am of the opinion that the first heart transplant was not a great medical breakthrough and certainly not a major scientific discovery of our century. I think that finding the structures of DNA was a much greater achievement for medical science.

> *I threw the gloves which I had used for the first heart transplant operation into the dustbin. Later someone offered me $50,000 for them.*

Perhaps this all sounds a bit too modest, but there is evidence that I didn't think any differently then than I do today. The night the big operation was planned I had not given any orders to prepare for anything special. I had not informed the hospital administration, nor did I think about taking photos of the operation to document one of the medical events of the century. For me the first heart transplant was nothing but the first clinical introduction of a new surgical technique. It was something we had already practiced many times, nothing really magic.

It was an error of judgment which I would soon regret. Only a few weeks after that historic night of December 3, 1967 a French company offered me $50,000 (!) for the surgical gloves I had worn during the operation. Fool that I was, I had thrown them away after the operation.

Much as I have since regretted that lost opportunity, I would like to say that I have never been a physician who was interested in becoming wealthy. Among the thousands of people I have given medical attention to, not one has ever had to pay me even a dollar.

Today I survive on a $700-a-month pension.

I was never in it for the money. I once even turned down a very good opportunity to earn millions. It was at the beginning of the seventies at the New Orleans airport. I was between flights on my way home to South Africa. A passenger came up to me and immediately came to the point: "Excuse me, professor, for taking the liberty of speaking to you directly, but I recognized you and would like to make you an offer. Come to my office and let me draw up a contract for you. I would like to act as your manager. You will never regret this."

I was quite bemused by this gentleman and his offer. I cordially thanked him – and turned him down. I could not quite reconcile the offer with my professional dignity. Besides, what kind of big business could this gentleman have wanted to do with me? His name was not known to me at the time; I later learned he was Mark McCormick, who has since become one of the world's most successful managers and has a great many international stars – especially sports stars – under contract.

I can honestly say that it was my calling to become a doctor. I was born in 1922, one of four children, in the small South African town of Beaufort West. The roots of my family on my father's side can be traced to Cologne in Germany, and on my mother's side to France. My mother's ancestors were Huguenots. My father worked as a missionary in Beaufort West and my mother was the organist at the local church. I always wanted to be a doctor, something that could certainly not be taken for granted since we were not very well off.

I studied medicine with a certain feeling of panic. I was always afraid of failing one of my exams, as my family could hardly afford the expensive tuition. I will never forget the day my eldest brother failed an exam. It was a virtual tragedy for the family; for days we all reacted as though we had lost a good friend.

The relationship among the siblings was not as close as might be supposed. But we all got on well enough with one another and helped each other when we could. My brother Marius assisted me during my first heart transplant. Today he is retired and lives near Cape Town. We talk occasionally on the phone, but only see each other about once a year.

I always wanted to be a doctor because I wanted to help people. I was always very goal-oriented and ambitious. I never thought of these as bad qualities. I put great effort into my studies. Not being able to afford a car, I walked the four miles to the university in Cape Town every day.

I passed all my exams, some with honors, and upon graduating as a doctor I received a scholarship to continue my studies in the United States. By that time I had decided I was going to be a surgeon specializing in the heart. I went to the University of Minnesota in Minneapolis. It was there that I saw the first open heart operation using a heart–lung machine. How primitive everything was back then, and how mistaken the theories!

To me it appears so simple today to prevent a heart attack.

Just how easy is the subject of this book.

Nutrition

1 Forget About Diets

The bad news: diets can make you fat, sick, depressive. The good news: you don't have to diet to lose weight.

I have always been a bit privileged in my life. I have never been overweight and never needed to go on a diet. The most weight I ever had to carry around with me was 180 pounds, but that was years ago. Currently I weigh 165 pounds, and since I am 6 feet tall I would consider myself on the thin side.

I think my weight has to do with my lifestyle and probably a little with my genes. My father was thin and my mother as well. Actually there was never anyone in my family who had problems with weight.

> *My mother gave me the best dieting idea in the world: "Stop eating when you're still hungry."*

I have always eaten in moderation and never had to force myself to eat in a healthy way. I like fruit and vegetables because we grew them in our own garden. However, I never put myself under pressure. If I have an appetite for meat, I will eat meat. Sometimes I have a craving for cakes because I certainly have a sweet tooth. Yet, regardless of what I eat, I always remember what my mother used to say: "Stop eating while you're still hungry." Nothing can be more effective for keeping thin than this little piece of wisdom.

Dieting is seldom done for health reasons; it is usually done for the sake of appearance. I don't think I have ever met a person who wanted to lose weight to relieve the pressure on his spinal column, to improve his liver functions, or to look after his heart. Everyone wanted to lose weight in order to look better and more attractive. Television programs and magazines show us everyday that thin people are loved more, have more success, and simply just do better in life. Young women who model have to be thin, even skinny.

Reality, however, can no longer keep up with television. Even though we are constantly bombarded with new diet schemes, there have never been so many overweight people in the industrialized nations.

Obesity will be the greatest health problem of the 21st century.

- Every third American is overweight, one in five is grossly overweight – that is, fat.
- 10 million Germans are too fat. An increasing number of children are also overweight.
- Obesity and the resulting illnesses cost the American medical system $50 billion a year.
- Individual costs are exploding as well. An overweight person spends 25% more on health care, an obese person 44% more than the average person.
- Many experts believe obesity will be the biggest health problem of the 21st century.

A friend of mine has gained quite a bit of weight in recent years. When I asked him why he hadn't tried to diet, he answered jokingly: "One would not be enough for me. I would need at least two diets." He's right, in a way: his chances of success would not increase if he tried 10 or 20 diet plans. It has been proved that virtually all who try to lose pound by pound regain their original weight within five years. Some gain even more.

There is a simple explanation for this. During dieting the body adapts to the new situation and the metabolism is lowered, because, as the American nutritional specialist Jack Goppel put it:

4

"the body cannot know if you're in the process of losing weight or on the verge of starving." The result is that less energy is used up because the body tries to pace itself – adapting to the new situation. At some point the diet is finished and it's back to the usual eating habits. But the body is still in its austerity mode. Quickly, much faster than you were able to lose the pounds, they're back again. After dieting you're soon back to square one and may end up even worse off than that.

> Every second woman has tried to diet at least once. Every second teenager wants to lose weight.

Despite limited chances of success, the dieting obsession is affecting an increasing number of people. This is confirmed by a research study done by the German Society for Nutrition:

- Only one in four Germans is happy with his/her figure.
- One in two German women have tried dieting at least once.
- Fifty percent of all teenagers want to lose weight.
- Virtually no one manages to lose weight and keep it off.

People who try repeatedly to attain their ideal weight through dieting and do not achieve their goal see themselves as failures. Because almost no one knows that diets cannot work, everyone blames him- or herself. The thought that something must be done and that the next diet might be the solution makes dieting a big business. Diet schemes in Germany have a turnover far in excess of 100 million marks.

Diets not only make you fat and depressive, they also make you sick. According to an American research study, weight-obsessed individuals are twice as likely to contract heart disease as the national average. The risk of diabetes is five times as high.

A research survey in Florida found that 23% of those who regularly dieted complained of heart trouble. Of those in the survey who never dieted, only about 11% complained of heart problems.

> He who stays hungry not only leaves himself with nothing to chew on – he can jeopardize what he has to chew with: his teeth.

Particularly problematic are crash diets, in which the dieter tries to lose weight very rapidly. They burden the organism more than common diets. In the opinion of the American Dental Association, crash diets can even be harmful to teeth and gums. Vegetarian diets, above all, frequently lead to deficits in calcium, Vitamins D and B_{12}, and protein, all of which play an important role in keeping the teeth and gums healthy.

Diets Lead to Eating Disorders

More frequently diets are the direct cause of another problem: according to German nutritional experts, 90% of people who have tried more than four diets are to some degree prone to eating disorders. Never before in Germany have there been so many cases of anorexia and bulimia as there are today.

But there is no reason to give up hope of losing weight. Every person has the potential to lose it and keep it off. And it is really quite simple. But you must forget about diets if you want to lose weight. Think about your life for 10 minutes and start making changes *there*, not with the food you eat. How often do you eat because you want to reward yourself? How often do you eat something even though you're not hungry – maybe just because everyone else is eating? And what about exercise in your daily routine?

Losing weight is so simple. Eighty percent of all those who are overweight do not need a diet plan at all in order to lose weight. Make a few changes in your lifestyle and you're on course. At the end of this chapter I will reveal a few tricks on how to lose weight without having to make too many sacrifices in the quality of your life.

Weight reduction is done in small steps. The quicker the fix, the sooner you will have regained whatever it was you managed to shake off. Here is how to go about real weight-reduction in three steps.

Step 1 Establish whether you need to lose weight at all.
Step 2 Check to see what is making you fat. What are you eating?
Step 3 Accept the fact that weight reduction without exercise cannot work.

First and foremost: throw your bathroom scales away.

There are many ways to start a diet. One of the best ways to start is to throw your bathroom scales into the garbage. Nothing is more detrimental to losing weight than the daily pilgrimage to the scales. The scales promote a few days of euphoria because you have lost 2 or 3 pounds (sadly, mostly water and very little fat). They will, however, provoke great frustration within a week – at the point where the scales refuse to show a weight loss even though you're living on bread and water.

A good weight-reduction programme is always long term and has nothing to do with what your scales say. The best way to lose weight is to find out exactly what kind of shape you're in. To establish this, there are various possibilities.

- The Broca-Index. For years this was the ultimate guideline. Height in centimetres minus 100 was the basis for establishing the weight norm. For example, a woman measuring 155 cm (approx 5 ft.) would subtract 100 to come up with the weight of 55 kg (about 120 pounds).
- The Feel-Good Index. Many people try to lose pounds in order to reach their ideal weight, even though this is not necessary. Therefore a new guideline was created. Normal weight according to Broca, and up to 10% above or below that weight, became acceptable as normal. This is the area in which most people feel comfortable.
- The Body-Mass Index. But no two people are alike, so the body mass index (BMI) was developed in the United States. The formula is as follows: body weight in kilograms divided by height in metres squared. Let's use me as an example. I am 1 metre 80 centimetres tall and weigh 75 kilograms. 1.80 squared is 3.24. 75 kilos divided by 3.24 is 23.1. Therefore my BMI is 23.1, in the so-called green area. A level above 25 means "slightly overweight" and more than 30 "extremely overweight."

But the BMI also has its weak points. Take the Austrian skier Herman Maier, for example – a model athlete who is 1 metre 90 cm tall. During the final heated weeks of the skiing World Cup he weighed 96 kilos. At this weight he reached a BMI of 26.6 and would therefore be considered slightly overweight. However, no one would ever have considered him too "chubby."

If all our measuring methods have their weak points, who can tell us what is right and healthy? Our own body. The greatest mistake made in most diets is that they place the emphasis on weight alone. Much more important than the number of pounds we carry around with us is the share of body fat. Fat tissue stores calories, muscles burn them. A sensible diet, therefore, has to ensure that the body fat amount is reduced while simultaneously building muscle. This is the reason why a diet without exercise is something for the garbage can. Exercises or sport help to stimulate the metabolism; weight-loss diets do the opposite. When you become active your body suddenly stops storing fat and begins to burn it – you begin to lose weight.

> *The simple mechanism of a sensible diet: you have to burn fat and build muscle.*

Your body fat percentage can easily be tested. Jump up and down naked in front of a mirror. If your skin is flapping about as if you were wearing a diving suit five times too big, then you are obviously too fat. Somewhat more accurate readings can be derived from a measuring device called a *caliper*, available in virtually every well-stocked sporting goods store. It has the shape of pliers which you can apply on your stomach or upper arms, creating a kind of fold that can be measured. Women should have a body fat level less than 22% and men should be under 17%.

My Three Weight-reduction Rules

OK, now you know that you have a few excess pounds. But what do you do? Above all, don't force yourself to give anything up. Let's say you like desserts. Think about what would happen if you eliminated sweets completely from your diet plan. You would not be able to think about anything else all day. Go ahead, eat some chocolate if you feel like it. You will soon see that you will eat only a few pieces and no longer devour the whole bar.

> *Rule 1: Deny yourself nothing.*

This is the crucial point. A weight-loss plan filled with "do nots" is not worth very much. Of course you can manage to eat mainly fruit and salads for a week. But to keep your weight you have to do it for the rest of your life. Honestly, who really wants to be a rabbit?

> *Rule 2: Use a nutritional plan to help you attain your ideal weight and remain there.*

This plan cannot be something abstract. It has to fit into your life and integrate itself. That is the reason why I do not like the words "dieting" or "slimming." Both mean "I'm only doing something over a short period of time." But a *nutrition plan* should be for life.

Finally, however, I want to give you the most important rule of weight loss:

> *Rule 3: Eat less.*

Even a small reduction in overall intake is usually sufficient. Does that sound simple? It is! Take the following 10 bits of advice to heart (!) and remember what my mother said: "Stop eating while you are still hungry."

> *Don't make a cult of your diet. Weight reduction is really a very simple process.*

Barnard Tips for a Healthy Heart
Slim without Fasting: The 10 Best Rules

1 **Be wary of dieting.**
   Most get-thin-quick diet programs only reduce the size of your wallet.
2 **Don't count calories.**
   Be honest, were you that good at maths at school?

3 Use your common sense.

Losing weight takes time. Attaining a bikini figure in two weeks only works in magazines.

4 Don't eat everything on your plate.

Your parents are probably very nice people, but not all their advice still applies now you are grown up.

5 Play tricks on your stomach.

Eat some noodle or tomato soup before the main course. Immediately you will eat less of it.

6 Eat more often.

Not eating for 12 hours and then raiding the refrigerator is no way to lose weight.

7 Take some time to contemplate.

Think about what you have eaten in the last 48 hours. You will be surprised.

8 Train yourself.

A healthy diet is like jogging. Practice a few times and it will come naturally.

9 Don't force yourself to give up anything.

If you love ice cream, go right ahead. You don't have to eat it every day.

10 No radical changes, please.

You don't all of a sudden put diesel fuel instead of gas in your car.

2 | Eat the Right Fat

Fat is back: eating butter and drinking milk
– in the right amounts – can be good for the heart.

I know of no other form of nutrition that has a worse image than fat. I always hear that fat makes us overweight and age before our time, clogs up our arteries, and serves as a precursor to cancer. The assurance that food is low in fat or without fat immediately makes it healthy in the eyes of many. Anyone eating fat, on the other hand, is an unrepentant fool, someone who is slowly eating him- or herself to death.

I don't like fat. I don't like the taste of it in my mouth. During my childhood at home we very rarely had meat with a meal. My father did not like it very much. Even today I can get by without a steak or pork chops. At most I eat meat only twice a week. But even here I am a bit of a surgeon; I cut away the fat from the lean portion of the meat.

> With fat intake it is not only a question of quantity but also of quality.

Today many people are doing the same thing I am. They don't eat fat. However it's not because they don't like it but rather because they have been told it will make them fat. According to an increasing number of nutritional experts, particularly in the United States, this is not necessarily the case. For years now, more and more products which are low in fat are being sold in super-markets. But Americans have nonetheless never been as fat as today.

This lies partly in the fact that we're cheating. We are, of course, eating much more today than 20 or 30 years ago. We don't have a bad conscience about it either, because we feel it isn't fat, after all, only low-fat yogurt along with a can of Diet Coke. Naturally fat still plays a definitive role in our being thin or overweight. But as the *New England Journal of Medicine* reported, "the decisive factor is not how much fat you eat, but the kind of fat you eat."

Fat is necessary for our bodies. It carries out an array of important functions:

- Fat gives us energy.
- Fat provides us with vitamins.
- Fat gives food its taste.
- Fat is an important building block for cells.
- Fat is a raw material for hormones and other regulatory substances in the body.

Without a doubt we all eat too much fat. We eat substantial meals, partly for historic reasons. In times of food shortages, as in Europe during and after the Second World War, fat played an absolutely vital role in nutrition. Fat filled and satisfied those who could get it. Those who had to do hard physical work got their energy from fat. Not without reason do we still speak of a "hearty meal," meaning that the meal is large, very satisfying, and certainly not without fat.

Times have quickly changed, but our eating habits have not quite kept pace. Only very few people today are engaged in hard physical work. Most people sit in cars, offices, and in the evening at home in front of the television. This means that a person now needs less fat than 30 or 40 years ago. Yet in Germany, for example, people take in 120 grams (approximately half a pound) of fat a day – almost double what they really need.

But that is not the only thing wrong with our current eating habits: most of the fat we eat is particularly unhealthy.

All fats have the same basic structure. A few simple differences are decisive in determining if it is good or bad for us. Fat consists of molecules and fatty acids. The framework of these fatty acids consists of carbon atoms which in turn combine with hydrogen atoms. If each carbon atom finds a hydrogen atom, then we speak of *saturated* fats. If a few of the carbon atoms remain single, we term these *unsaturated* fats.

> *Fat – in our time this simple food has become a science.*

It is important to know this because these terms are increasingly being used when speaking of fat. I have put together some of the most essential medical terms concerning fat so that you can understand what nutritional experts are talking about. However, my tip is, don't get hung up on technical terms. The more naturally you deal with fat, the fewer problems you will have with it.

THE LITTLE ABC OF FAT
The Most Important Terms and What They Mean
SATURATED FATS

These are mainly found in animal products such as meat, butter, eggs, cheese, and lard. Up until recently saturated fats were considered the devil incarnate. Today many nutrition experts are far less adamant about this. It is still considered a fact that saturated fats can foster the "bad cholesterol" (LDL) in the blood. But certain foods that used to be on the "forbidden list" are now considered healthy.

Among these are nuts and even butter, both of which provide valuable vitamins for the body. So it's safe to say that unless you really overdo it, saturated fats are not going to significantly raise your risk of arteriosclerosis.

MONOUNSATURATED FATS

These appear to be the true winners of the ongoing "fats" discussion. They reduce the "bad cholesterol" (LDL). Simple unsaturated fats can be found in olive oil, rapeseed oil, hemp oil, peanuts, poultry, and avocados. Olive oil is frequently given as a reason for the low incidence of heart attacks suffered by the indigenous people of the Mediterranean.

> *Monounsaturated fats are healthy. Olive or hemp oil, avocados, and peanuts are rich in these fats.*

POLYUNSATURATED FATS

These can be found in fish fat, sunflower oil, rapeseed oil, and soya, and for many years they were the darling of the food industry because of their reported positive effects on cholesterol levels. Today one sees the situation somewhat differently. Multiple unsaturated fats reduce not only the "bad" but the "good" cholesterol as well. Too much can be considered unhealthy.

LINOLEIC ACIDS

These are a special type of unsaturated fat. Laboratory tests on animals have raised speculation that the so-called conjugated linoleic acids can serve as protection against cancer and heart attacks. Curiously enough, linoleic acids are contained in produce that for many years was not considered particularly healthy: cheese, butter – and particularly milk. An increasing number of nutritionists are putting skimmed milk back on their recommended lists. The classic books on nutrition are celebrating a comeback.

ESSENTIAL FATTY ACIDS

The best known of these are the Omega 6 fatty acids and the Omega 3 fatty acids. We absorb the Omega 6 fatty acids through our regular diet, but we are lacking in the intake of Omega 3 fatty acids. We don't eat enough fatty fish (salmon, herring, mackerel), nuts, linseed, or green vegetables such as leeks and cabbage. Salad, too, is rich in Omega 3 fatty acids. By not eating enough food containing Omega 3 fatty acids we miss out on the protection they provide against heart attacks by thinning out the blood, and against diabetes – one of the biggest risk factors of heart and circulation diseases.

TRANS-FATTY ACIDS

These can be found in red meat, margarine, cookies, and many frozen foods, particularly in french fries and puff pastry. Trans-fatty acids have continually gained in importance in the food in-dustry over the past years. The hardening process of unsaturated fats creates them. Trans-fatty acids are increasingly coming under suspicion of heightening the risk of cancer and arteriosclerosis. A Harvard University study concluded that a person reducing their trans-fatty acid intake by only 4 grams a day cuts the risk of a heart attack in half

> *Eat balanced meals, put your main emphasis on vegetables and fruit. Then you won't be stressed by fat.*

Perhaps the biggest problem we have with fat today is the lack of perspective. No wonder, considering all the terms that we hear every day: unsaturated fats, Omega fatty acids, trans-fatty acids, etc. How can anyone not professionally involved with the subject be able to differentiate all the terms and know what's good? In the supermarkets the traditional marketing principle has never had more validity: "A person doesn't buy what he needs but what he knows."

But how does one recognize fat? It's practically impossible. Two-thirds of all the fat we eat is well hidden. We eat it with sausages, pizza, nuts, and even avocados. One chocolate bar and 100 grams of fat – and you have gone over the daily limit.

That is the reason why I have only one tip on the subject: don't succumb to fat stress. No one can work out his or her daily fat intake requirement using a chart. No one has enough time to decipher the chemical contents of a food product. I will only give you three simple rules for dealing with fat:

1 Eat a balanced diet. If the food mix is right then your fat intake will be OK.
2 Fall in love with fresh fruit and vegetables. Anyone enjoying a good range of these will not have problems with fat intake.
3 Use high-quality oils. Don't be confused by the array of names in the supermarket. The best quality in cold-pressed olive oil must now, according to new guidelines set by the European Union, be identified as "Native olive oil extra." Number two according to the new guidelines is "Native olive oil." Everything else is not worth the money despite the appealing packaging or brand name.

A new alternative to olive oil is hemp oil. In former times hemp was a valuable raw material. For a period of time in the United States it was used in the production of automobiles. They turned out to be so resilient that no one could make any money from them. Now hemp is making a comeback on another front: as oil. According to a German study, hemp oil has an unusually high amount of unsaturated fats, namely 90%. Particularly high is the portion of linoleic acids which are thought to protect against heart attacks.

> *Hemp oil is the Middle Europeans' answer to the olive oil of Italy and Greece.*

Barnard Tips for a Healthy Heart
The 10 Best Tricks for Dealing with Fat

1 **Variety is the spice of life.**
   Eat a good mix of fruits and vegetables. If you do this you can forget about fat-reduction pills.

2 **Take exercise, play sport.**
   Have you sinned with an overabundance of french fries? Then atone for it by swimming or jogging.

3 **Don't re-use oils.**
   Oil should be thrown out after use.

4 **Don't cut down too fast.**
   You cannot trick your body. If you eat light, it will ask for two portions.

5 **Stay alert.**
   Fat can be hidden anywhere, especially in pastries, pies, alcohol, nuts, etc.

6 **Look for quality.**
   The best quality oil in the supermarket carries the EU marking "Native oil extra."

7 **Treat your oil with care.**
   Don't buy large amounts and be sure to store in a dark place. Good oil is very sensitive.

8 **Down with fat.**

Don't breathe easy too early. Naturally you're eating too much per day – go easy on your intake.

9 **Try a few alternatives.**

How about hemp oil? Tastes good and contains many unsaturated fatty acids.

10 **Fats make you sexy.**

Laboratory tests with animals have shown: eating a low-fat diet is detrimental to the sex drive.

3 Drink Red Wine

You won't believe it but it's true.
A person drinking two glasses of
red wine a day is helping his heart.

I have always found the discussion about this somewhat strange. The whole world points a finger at cigarettes and billions are spent on anti-smoking campaigns, but our worst enemy is actually alcohol. It can damage the whole body: brain, heart, liver, and stomach. You most likely won't cause a traffic accident because of smoking and you probably won't hit your wife because you have smoked a cigarette, but both can occur as a result of peering a bit too deeply into the bottle. On the other hand, what is it about wine, beer, and other alcoholic beverages that all of a sudden they are being treated like medicine? Well, they can keep you healthy and lengthen your life. No more, no less.

> *Alcohol plays the role of Dr. Jekyll and Mr. Hyde. It is a killer, but it can also promote our health.*

I sometimes drink alcohol. Not every day and not regularly. I mainly drink at restaurants and very rarely at home. I am not a beer drinker and I don't like hard liquor; I prefer wine. I used to drink white wine, but because of my arthritis I switched to red.

I never drank wine to stay healthy. I drank it because I enjoyed it. For me that is the essential point. Drinking alcohol is not a sport. When you go to a fitness centre for the first time and get on a stationary bike, you will probably manage about 10 minutes. After a week it's probably 15 minutes and after a month 30 minutes. This is something you should never try with alcohol – consumption should always be in moderation. Used properly it can serve as medication, taking it incorrectly changes it to poison.

Curiously, most of the positive effects of moderate alcohol consumption have been known for a long time. Despite this, the medical community refused for decades to confirm officially the positive effects of alcohol on the heart. The reason is clear: in Germany alone more than 2.5 million people are alcoholics. Many medical scientists believe that this number would increase dramatically if wine were officially declared a form of medicine.

This attitude has changed in the meantime, due to the fact that more than 60 reliable research studies from around the world – from the USA to China – have established the positive effects on the circulatory system of red wine in particular. Currently the accepted positive effects of red wine are as follows:

- It's good for the blood.
- It can protect against arteriosclerosis.
- It has positive effects on cholesterol levels in the body.
- It helps control the effects of stress.
- It enhances the body's immune system.

David Goldberg, doctor and biochemist at the University of Toronto, states: "If every North American would drink two glasses of red wine every day, heart disease would be reduced by 40% and $40 billion in medical costs could be saved every year."

The first evidence of the positive effects of alcohol on health was discovered very early. Aristotle wrote: "He who knocks on the door of the muses bearing no wine will receive no reply." Caesar let his soldiers drink wine before going on a campaign in order to prevent intestinal illnesses. In the Bible it says: "Do not drink water any longer but take some wine to thee for the sake of thy stomach and because thou art ill often."

It took almost 2,000 years before we were again openly urged to drink wine for the sake of our health. On May 5, 1995 the respected *British Medical Journal* published a study undertaken in

Copenhagen, Denmark that made headlines around the world. The Danish doctor Martin Gronbaek and his team recorded and analysed the lifestyles of 13,000 people for 12 years. His conclusion: a person drinking wine regularly reduces the probability of dying from a heart attack by 60%.

The publication of the results of the study created a sensation. Suddenly dozens of previous studies were remembered which had come to similar conclusions:

- In 1926 the American biologist Raymond Pearl discovered that moderate alcohol consumption was linked to a lower risk of heart attack. A person drinking two to three glasses of wine a day would reduce his chances of getting a heart attack by 40%.
- In a large-scale study done in the 1970s, the Californian cardiologist Dr. Arthur Klatsky was able to confirm that moderate alcohol consumption can reduce the risk of heart attacks.
- In 1990 the American Cancer Society published findings based on the medical profiles of 277,000 men. Once again the results were similar: one alcoholic drink a day reduces the risk of heart disease by 25%.

> *Drinking red wine can reduce the risk of a heart attack by 60 percent.*

Until the Danish study it was unclear which alcohol provided the biggest positive effect. Gronbeak was the first to confirm reliably ˙iest form of alcohol. Beer lovers who drink ˙manage to reduce their chances of a heart was found to have no positive effects on other diseases such as cancer. Individuals drinking strong alcoholic beverages such as whiskey or other hard liquors had practically no medical advantages when compared to teetotallers.

> *Wine is the outright winner. Beer does nothing against cancer, hard liquor has practically no medical advantage.*

Attitudes have changed. Since the publication of the Danish findings an increasing number of red wine's positive characteristics have been uncovered:

- Wine is good for the heart. Even the heart specialists of the respected American College of Cardiology recommend drinking a glass of red regularly. By doing this, one in two Americans could reduce the risk of a heart attack.
- Red wine can serve as preventive protection. A French study concluded that moderate consumption of red wine could also be useful after suffering a heart attack, and that – especially in combination with a Mediterranean-style diet (lots of fish, fresh fruit and vegetables, and high-quality oils) – it can help prevent a second heart attack.
- Wine can protect against strokes. The Copenhagen Institute for Preventive Medicine was able to find evidence that moderate wine consumption can perceptibly reduce the risk of a stroke. A person drinking a glass a day reduces his or her chances of having a stroke by 32%.
- Wine contains substances such as quercetin, resveratrol, and catechin. These secondary plant substances are mostly absorbed by the wine during storage in kegs, but can be found in must and in grape skin as well. Secondary plant substances have an anti-oxidizing effect. Stated simply, they prevent the arteries from rusting.
- According to a study done at Harvard University, alcohol favors an enzyme which plays a central role in dissolving dangerous clots in the blood. Therefore it can help in preventing thromboses and heart attacks.
- Consumed as an aperitif, wine stimulates the development of the gastrin hormone, which plays an important role in the digestive process.
- A research study in Wales found that red wine has the best effects on men between the ages of 55 and 64. In this age group the risk of a heart attack is particularly high.
- The German Society for the Prevention and Rehabilitation of Heart and Circulatory Diseases concluded that wine has positive effects on blood clotting. Alcohol can also raise the

levels of the "good cholesterol" HDL and lower the "bad cholesterol" LDL. Higher levels of HDL prevent deposits from forming on the blood vessel walls.

- Moderate consumption of alcohol can reduce stress, provide relief from sleep disorders, and positively influence your overall well-being.

Wine is one of the pleasures of life – and it helps you relax and sleep well.

Red wine has an additional asset that cannot be easily measured scientifically: it serves the pleasure principle. It helps us relax in a pleasant atmosphere, perhaps in the evening when we want to settle down and get cosy, or when we want to savor a particularly good meal. We enjoy – and therefore, certainly in the spirit of a healthy heart – we get more out of life.

Barnard Tips for a Healthy Heart
Ten Ways to Use the Power of Wine

1 **Consume in moderation.**
   Two glasses of red wine a day are OK. More is a competition.
2 **It's a pleasure.**
   It's a kind of luxury – a personal luxury you prescribe for yourself.
3 **Drink regularly.**
   A heart assassin: abstinence for five days and then over-consumption and hangover time at weekends.
4 **Don't force yourself to drink.**
   If you don't like the taste of alcohol then don't drink it.
5 **Think about alternatives.**
   Grape and elderberry juice are almost as good as wine, but only almost.
6 **Buy quality.**
   Better quality red wine usually has the higher quality substances.

7 Wine is your friend.

It relaxes you, helps you sleep, and it oils the wheels of socializing.

8 Wine is your enemy.

First it washes away your worries, but then you get carried away.

9 Wine is not a cure-all.

It cannot alter the consequences of smoking too much or not exercising enough.

10 Wine is like sex.

Enjoy it, but don't try to understand it.

4 Live Heartily

Ten simple tricks for doing something
for your heart every day – while
shopping or during a meal.

I not only learned to handle a scalpel in my life; I can also do
quite well with a kitchen knife. This is partly due to the fact that
for a few years I owned a restaurant in South Africa. It did quite
well, and once I even had to play chef for a whole evening. My
Belgian maitre d' had served spoiled fish and, after an angry exchange of words with me, he left the restaurant in a huff. So I had
no choice but to man the pots and pans myself. Amazingly enough
I heard no complaints. The place was packed the whole evening.
Perhaps it was due to my good cooking or perhaps to the novelty of
seeing a heart surgeon sweating away in the kitchen.

I don't want to lay down any rules on how you should go about
preparing a meal, and certainly not on what kind of restaurant you
should avoid. But just read what follows and you will see that
sometimes it can be quite easy to do something for your heart.

Trick 1. Buy Often

Much has become so simple. Once a week everyone gets in the car
and heads off to the supermarket. Then it's buy, buy, buy as if there
were no tomorrow. Plenty of fruit and vegetables are purchased –
after all, we're living a healthy lifestyle. I want to tell you once and
for all: forget it! Sure, it's practical to go shopping for groceries

once for the whole week. But you're not helping your body or your heart. Why? Because even in the best refrigerator in the world the most valuable ingredients of fruit and vegetables are gone after a few days. Salad, for instance, has a half-life of two days, after which 50% of the vitamin C content is gone. It's not much different with spinach, chard or cabbage. Oxygen, heat, light, and dampness all have negative effects on food products.

> *Don't leave fruit and vegetables in the refrigerator too long. They lose vitamins.*

I don't want to talk you out of going grocery shopping once a week. But at least try to buy fruit and vegetables as fresh as possible and, if you can, go to a farmer's market and buy it there.

Trick 2. Don't Shop When You're Hungry

This is one of the best tricks I know. It not only helps the heart, but is also easy on the wallet. Much of what we buy we don't really need. It just lies around our refrigerator for a while until it is spoiled and we have to throw it out. Try to recall the last time you went shopping. You went from shelf to shelf and thought about what great things you could make with each item you saw. This only happens when you go grocery shopping hungry. If you're full then it's not your stomach talking in the supermarket, but your mind.

Trick 3. Take a Break

Nowadays you can't just go into a supermarket and buy some yogurt, for instance. You end up standing in front of endless shelves filled with multitudes of colorful packages. On each package you discover countless names of chemical components you've never heard of. There are only two things you can do: be mad at your parents for not letting you study medicine, biology, or chemistry, or take a five-minute break. What can you do in these five minutes? Above all you can take a closer look at the packaging. You probably won't be able to make out all the components contained within (especially the chemical descriptions) but some things will appear familiar to you. Where does the item come from? What does it actually consist of? How high is the fat content? How high is the fruit content? How many calories (or kilojoules) does it have per 100 grams? Soon you will see that in order to get the most important information you don't need to have a degree in chemistry.

> *Confusing, perhaps, but instructive: read the labels.*

Trick 4. Live According to the Season

If you go into a supermarket today, no matter what time of year it is everything appears rich and colorful. You can get virtually every kind of vegetable and fruit throughout the year. But experience will tell you that strawberries don't grow when there is snow on the ground. Therefore the strawberries in the supermarket must be imported from somewhere. Fruit and vegetables that are imported usually have quite an odyssey behind them before they make it to our supermarkets. The extended transportation time and a synthetic ripening process pretty well guarantee that very little is left of the once proud vitamin package. However, there is a simple way to be on the safe side: only buy fresh fruit and vegetables that are in season in your region. For instance, strawberries in spring, peaches in summer and pears in early autumn.

> *To be on the safe side, buy fruit which grows in your area.*

Trick 5. Take Your Groceries for a Walk

Grocery shopping as a form of exercise? It is easily possible. Here are the simplest examples:

- The jogging exercise. You know the routine. You drive to the supermarket and all the parking spaces close to the entrance are full. But be happy, because just this situation will keep you moving. Park your car as far away from the entrance as possible and walk the rest of the way.

- The kneeling exercise. In supermarkets the products that are most likely to attract your attention are those placed at eye-level. One or two shelves below that you may very well find the same kind of product, possibly cheaper. So do some kneeling.
- The sprint exercise. There are many products in supermarkets which are usually located close by the tills. One quickly puts these into the trolley without thinking. Race past these, you very rarely need them.
- The lifting exercise. You know the problem. You come laden down with bottles to recycle and there is no one around to help. Well, time for some exercise. Lift the bottles out by yourself.
- The head-shaking exercise. The tills attract your children more than playgrounds. The reason? All the candies on display. Mostly they are too expensive and very sweet. If your children pester you to buy some, your reaction should be a vigorous shake of the head.

Trick 6. Be a Role Model

There is nothing that shapes our lives more than our home environment. How our parents let us grow up usually determines if we're successful, happy, and healthy in our lives. We derive many of our habits from our parents, in particular our eating habits. If eating was a family affair in your parents' house, then most likely you will adhere to this as well. If you grew up as I did, with plenty of fruit and vegetables in the house, then you will have them around for your children. Make it a virtue to be a role model when it comes to eating.

Trick 7. Eat According to Your Whims and Moods

Think about when you take a knife and fork in your hands. Is it when you're hungry or when everyone else is eating? It is one of the strangest habits we learn. Breakfast, lunch, and dinner are set for fixed times and we eat regardless of whether we feel like eating or not. It's time to stop this silly habit. Only eat when your body signals that it's hungry. This keeps you healthy and thin.

Trick 8. Restrict Yourself to Your Meals

Eating is a matter of concentration. If you are doing things while you're eating, you'll be distracted from your natural eating rhythm. Reading a newspaper is probably OK (albeit not very sociable) because turning the pages is such a chore that you automatically eat slowly. But hands and eyes off the TV, computer games, or anything similar.

This holds true for the office as well. Make it a rule never to eat at your desk, then you won't be tempted to look through a few reports or take a call.

> *You can't eat properly at the office. Intrusions, phone calls, etc. will just get in the way.*

Trick 9. Take Five Minutes Longer to Eat

Everywhere in the world fast food is booming. The revenue of traditional restaurants is decreasing while the fast food chains prosper. For 18 years now McDonald's has been Germany's biggest restaurant group. The 930 branches have an annual turnover of 3.8 billion German marks. The problem with fast food restaurants is not that they exist or what we eat there. I certainly don't want to rob you of your appetite for a hamburger. If it's mayonnaise and other calorie-laden extras you enjoy, then go ahead and eat them. Just don't do it very often. Not every day and not every week. Hamburgers won't kill you, but if they're part of your regular lifestyle then you should quickly rethink your situation. Above all, don't use the ease and availability as an excuse: "I don't have time to eat anything else."

Trick 10. Chew Properly

"Eat slowly, chew properly." Whose parents didn't get on their children's nerves with such admonishments? Two British researchers literally sank their teeth into the problem. They developed a computer program that perfectly simulates the chewing mechanism of humans. They were able to conclude the following:

- It is wrong not to chew enough. If you just gobble down your food, you will have more difficulty digesting it. A well-known fact.
- It is also wrong to chew too much. The stomach receives food in clumps called a bolus. If it is chewed too much the bolus falls apart and the stomach has real problems processing the food.

Use your natural instincts. Don't gobble your food, no one wants to take it away from you. But don't chew every piece of food 100 times. You're only wasting time and not helping your stomach one bit.

5 Eat Vitamins

Vitamins are the new superstars in medicine. They help soothe stress, prevent cancer, and protect the heart.

Elephants don't take vitamin pills. "That's understandable," you might say. "Where would they get them? Besides, elephants spend all their lives in nature and only eat natural foods."

That's true, but just consider for a minute what would happen if elephants started to live like people. They would go out and buy a microwave, a fridge, and a TV. They would delete plants from their daily diet and replace them with fast food. They would smoke and not exercise very much either. If the elephant in question would ask me, as a doctor, if it were necessary to take vitamin pills along with his normal diet, I would answer "yes."

We have a lifestyle that practically screams for more vitamins. But we are eating fewer foods that provide us with the necessary nutritional value. Our fruit and vegetables no longer come from our gardens or the farms in our region, but from all over the world. When they finally land in our stomach, very little is left over from those highly praised superstars: vitamins. You enjoy juicy strawberries and can never pass up the appealing carrots and deep green leaves of spinach at the supermarket. My suggestion: continue to eat as you have, but don't do it because you believe that you are getting enough vitamins. A few years ago a German magazine decided to investigate the real vitamin content of our food. The findings were sobering:

- In a span of 11 years the vitamins in our food products have somehow secretly managed to disappear. In 1985 100 grams of strawberries still had a vitamin C content of 60 milligrams. In 1996 it was only 13 milligrams. In order to obtain the recommended daily requirement of 75 milligrams of vitamin C we would have to eat almost five times as many strawberries as 11 years ago.
- The situation is similar with other fruit. In the same time span apples lost approximately 80% of their vitamin C content. Bananas lost 92% of their vitamin B_6 content and 94% of their folic acid.
- Vegetables are losers in the findings too. Spinach has 58% less vitamin C content and 59% less vitamin B_6. Broccoli lost 52% of its folic acid content and beans have lost 61% of their vitamin B_6 content.

What is the reason for this? Well, one reason is that nature does not let itself be tricked that easily. Fruit and vegetables are cultivated today and forced into synthetically created ripening processes which reduce the vitamin and mineral content. We are paying the price for fruit that is available throughout the year.

> *Scientists are still finding valuable new properties in vitamins.*

One thing is for sure: vitamins are an essential part of our diet. For a long time their value for the organism was underestimated. Now there is an increasing amount of evidence showing the positive effects of vitamins. Many research studies have confirmed that vitamins play an important role in therapy and a decisive role in preventing an array of illnesses: migraine, chronic inflammation of the liver, osteoporosis, arthritis, and even Alzheimer's disease are among the increasing number of illnesses being treated with vitamins. Even in cancer prevention there is hope of a breakthrough. Two major American studies give hope that with the correct vitamin dose the cancer death rate can be dramatically reduced.

However, vitamins can do most for the heart. They provide our body with weapons to battle the so-called oxidation process.

What is happening inside us? Well, every day our metabolism produces various by-products, which in medical circles are called free radicals. The body sees these molecules in two ways. They are a bit like Dr. Jekyll and Mr. Hyde. As Dr. Jekyll they help us fight infections and destroy dangerous bacteria. As Mr. Hyde they also attack healthy tissue and cause great damage.

> *Free radicals can become the enemy of the body. Vitamins fight them off.*

This is the time for the antioxidants to come into the picture. They are a virtual army of nutrients, enzymes, and other chemical substances that can protect the body from oxidation. Oxidation is a process that occurs in nature millions of times. One only has to think of rusting nails: the iron has been oxidized. Antioxidants see to it that nothing "rusts" in us. Three vitamins lead the battle against this dangerous enemy: C, E, and betacarotene (a pro-vitamin, an early stage of vitamin A).

Free radicals are continuously produced in our body. However, the development of these dangerous molecules can be fostered by ozone, tobacco smoke, drinking large amounts of alcohol, heavy metal contamination, pollution, environmentally dangerous substances, and exposure to radiation or stress. An overdose of free radicals can weaken the heart muscles and reduce their output. An overdose of free radicals does this by damaging various structures of the heart muscle such as the membrane, which is the cell wall of the heart muscle, the enzymes in the heart cell, or even the structure of the cell core with its genetic material. The antioxidants serve as the body's police force, keeping the wild antics of the free radicals in check. However, where there are no police there can be no order.

> *Free radicals and oxygen: a love story which can have serious consequences for the body.*

Free radicals play a decisive role in arteriosclerosis, the much talked about hardening of the arteries. What happens? In your body two things are magically attracted to each other: oxygen and fat. If they become lovers, then oxidation takes place. The fat starts to spoil and so-called peroxides develop, a particularly dangerous form of free radicals. These again can best be fought by the army of antioxidants – vitamins C, E, and betacarotene.

Not all fats immediately fall for oxygen. Very simple unsaturated fats such as those found in olive oil remain relatively "cool" towards oxygen. This may be one of the reasons why people in countries where a great deal of olive oil is used – like France and Greece – have a lower incidence of heart ailments.

> *Our body has no problem with free radicals – if we support it.*

There is no reason to panic. Our body can deal quite well with free radicals – if we assist it. There are three ways to supply the antioxidant army with the right weaponry:

1 Eat as many vegetables and as much fruit as you can stuff inside yourself. Experts estimate that one would have to eat up to five balanced meals a day to supply the antioxidant army with enough vitamins. Your nutritional mix could consist of milk, nuts, strawberries, leafy vegetables, or potatoes – and this five times a day. The problem with this – apart from the fact that our food is becoming less and less "valuable" – is that we seldom eat the balanced meals our bodies actually require.
2 Try to avoid food products that can release a large amount of free radicals in your body. These would be saturated fats and trans-fatty acids. Here, too, there is a problem: trans-fatty acids develop during industrial food processing. They lie dormant in many food products (from cookies to margarine) without our being able to recognize them.
3 You supplement your diet with an antioxidant cocktail, a special kind of multi-vitamin preparation. Naturally you can take vitamins individually, but it is very difficult to diagnose which nutrients you're actually missing. Multi-vitamin preparations do not pose the danger of being "overdosed" because they consist of a balanced mix of vitamins, minerals, trace elements, and nutrients.

> *The body cannot manufacture its own vitamins (exception: vitamin D). Vitamins must be ingested.*

THE VITAMIN GUIDE
An Overview of the Most Important Vitamins

Vitamin	Effects	Main Sources	Daily Dose
A (retinol)	Regulates the splitting of cells, keeps the mucous membrane intact, produces male semen, important for the eyes	Found exclusively in animal products (butter, milk, cheese, liver)	0.9 mg (equivalent to 140 g of butter)
Pro-vitamin A (betacarotene)	Works as an antioxidant (fights free radicals)	Spinach, green cabbage, red peppers	2 mg (equivalent to 100 g of carrots)
B_1 (thiamin)	Important as a source of energy for carbohydrates	Wheat germ, nuts, pork	1.2 mg (45 g of peas)
B_2 (riboflavin)	Source of energy in fats and carbohydrates	Liver, linseed, eggs, cheese	1.6 mg (890 g of milk)
Niacin	Important for the metabolism, skin, brain	Poultry, liver, nuts, beans	17 mg (110 g of coffee beans)
B_6 (pyridoxine)	Important for the metabolism, muscles, hormones	Salmon, soya, rice, millet	1.7 mg (180 g of walnuts)
Folic acid	Important for cell splitting, red blood cells, nerves	Liver, spinach, endive	300 mg (250 g of nuts)
Pantothenic acid	Necessary for the production of cholesterins and hormones	Liver, eggs, lentils	6 mg (230 g of peanuts)

> *Spinach: what it lacks in iron it makes up in vitamin C.*

Vitamin	Effects	Main Sources	Daily Dose
B_{12} (cobalamin)	Important for blood production, sperm, nerves	Liver, herring, cheese, cottage cheese	3 mg (2 eggs)
C (ascorbic acid)	Antioxidant, important for immunity, hormones	Broccoli, strawberries, kiwi, potatoes	75 mg (120 g of a citrus fruit)
D (calciferol)	Regulates the calcium "household" of the body	Herring, salmon, avocado	5 mg (2 eggs)
E (tocopherol)	Has an antioxidant effect	Nuts and high-quality seed oils	12 mg (1 teaspoon of wheat germ oil)
H (biotin)	Important for the skin, hair and hormones	Liver, egg yolk, soya	100 mg (150 g of hazel nuts)
K (menachinon)	Important for the blood flow	Sauerkraut, broccoli, poultry	70 mg (25 g of spinach)

6 Eat with Passion

Don't let the killjoys and cranks spoil your
appetite. Continue to eat as your heart desires.

Eating has always been something special for me. I savor my
food. When I'm having a meal I want to sit at a nicely set table and
have plenty of time to enjoy my food. I belong to another generation. I really don't have much interest in fast food. Before I have a
quick bite standing, I'd rather eat nothing at all. However, I have
noticed that, particularly among children, fast food has an almost
magical appeal.

> *Rather than eat something quickly while standing up, I'd prefer to
> eat nothing at all.*

For us of the older generation, eating has a different value. My
father was poor and we were not faced with the daily decision of
eating a quick sandwich at home or going out to a luxury restaurant. That leaves a lasting impression.

I have always been very aware of what I eat. It hasn't been for
medical reasons, but because I have always enjoyed food too
much to consume it without taking the necessary time for a meal.

A few pages ago I tried to provide you with information concerning the positive effects of drinking red wine in moderation.
Perhaps you shook your head in disbelief because you couldn't
understand that alcohol, which many see as one of the most

dangerous and addictive drugs, can be good for anyone. But let's momentarily forget about the healthy contents of red wine. What then remains of the national drink of the French and the Spanish? The pure joy of life. Wine is a pleasurable luxury, just like good food. And people who can savor these things get more out of life.

What does eating mean to us today? Very often it is a negative experience. When we talk of food we speak of dieting, high cholesterol levels, fats that make us ill, and cancer-causing ingredients. We live with calorie charts, vitamin charts, mineral charts, and vital substance charts. We read about how the food industry is continually ruining our natural foods, and how farmers are maltreating their fields by spraying them with pesticides. After all this, how can eating still be fun? The pleasure of the past has turned into a burden.

But don't let yourself be carried away by all this commotion. Continue to enjoy your food, but above all, listen to your body. Most people still have a natural instinct for knowing what is good and what is bad for them. This instinct is sustained after trends and crazes have long gone. For many it came as no surprise that some natural food products, which had been blacklisted for years, all of a sudden had their reputation restored. The crusade against butter, eggs, chocolate, and coffee had taken on almost fanatical proportions. Now all of a sudden the vitamin content of butter is being praised. Eggs are no longer virtual cholesterol bombs, coffee is said to possess antioxidant powers, and chocolate is even considered a valuable ally in the battle against cancer.

> *Listen to your body, it knows what's good for you.*

For a long time a healthy diet had to do with sacrifices. If a person wanted to be slender and supple it meant clearing their plate of all their favorites and concentrating on selected foods which were frequently tasteless and charmless. Chefs actually tried to make appealing, colourful creations out of these boring ingredients, with only reasonable success.

But how could it work? How can one enjoy food if one constantly has to be afraid of it? What tastes good cannot be healthy, so the thinking went.

The End of Prohibition

A human being is a whole, not a nutritional machine that has to be fed only the right substances to function perfectly. A person also lives by his senses. Physicians know that enjoying life and having a positive outlook are important for a healthy body. And we are what we eat.

> *Eating "rules" play much too big a role in our lives.*

Don't fill your life with rules and prohibitions. Sure, we all eat too much fat, we eat too quickly, and our diets are unbalanced. But we don't do this with the intention of harming our bodies. We do it because we no longer deal naturally with food. Eating is no longer a reflex: "I am hungry, therefore I eat." Eating has much too high a priority in our lives. It is now a matter of the mind and no longer a matter of the stomach.

I'm not surprised that so many have problems with their weight and an increasing number of people have eating disorders. Over the past years eating has become a kind of enemy. All too often we have heard that bread, butter, eggs, meat, coffee, milk, and fat have no other purpose than to attack our bodies and harm us. How do you treat an enemy? You ignore him, you fight him, or you try to placate him. But you don't love him. That's the whole point: eating should be about love, lust and passion.

This does not mean you should have the license to eat indiscriminately. You should not tell yourself that steaks, pies, and french fries are good for you. Naturally you should take care to eat more fruit and vegetables and try to reduce consumption of synthetic fats. But don't declare war on your favorite foods, because there is no such thing as "healthy" or "unhealthy" food. There is only too much or too little. A glass of milk (particularly skimmed milk) a day is healthy, but try drinking three quarts and see what signals you get from your body. Most likely: too fat, too heavy.

> *Food is not only there to titillate the palate and the stomach, but the whole body, including the eyes.*

The secret of good eating is *variety*. A person who eats a balanced diet does not need a slimming plan, cholesterol charts, or fat-counters. A varied diet means having a broad spectrum to your nutritional mix; to eat everything that you like – in moderation.

Eat with all your senses. Do it like the Japanese or the Chinese: for them good food is not only dependent on taste. They also eat with their eyes. Anyone who has ever been to a Japanese restaurant knows that sushi or sashimi, two of the most renowned Japanese specialities, are never served alone on a tacky paper plate but are garnished with colourful vegetables on a wooden platter. Why? Because food is not only for your taste buds and your belly, but should be a pleasurable experience for the whole body.

Barnard Tips for a Healthy Heart

Ten Ways to Get More Pleasure Out of Eating

1 **Look forward to meals.**

   Be honest, is your life so much fun that you can forego this kind of enjoyment?

2 **Relax with your meal.**

   Forget your boss for half an hour, he's certainly not always thinking about you.

3 **Make a production out of your meal.**

   It doesn't always have to be candle-lit, but eating with style makes it more enjoyable.

4 **Eat with your eyes.**

   Remember your first date; you got all dressed up for that, didn't you?

5 **Think positive.**

   Healthy food can taste good. You only have to want it to.

6 **Don't think radical.**

   Changing your diet is OK, but don't overtax your body.

7 **Eat more.**

   Even more? Yes, more vitamins and minerals, possibly even nutritional supplements.

8 **Stay skeptical.**

   Not every idea concerning nutrition is a good one. Or do you believe everything you read in the papers?

9 Lie to your taste buds.

Hate eating vegetables? Drink them instead, as juices.

10 Don't force yourself to give things up.

Everything that is forbidden is tempting. At some point you give in, so don't put pressure on yourself always to be "good."

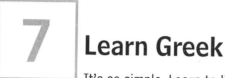

7 | Learn Greek

It's so simple. Learn to live like the people of Crete. Heart disease is practically unknown there.

Crete? Naturally you've heard of Crete, a Greek island in the Mediterranean. Perhaps you have even been there on holiday. You probably lay on the beach without a care in the world. Well, you probably needed the respite and that's as it should be, but I have to tell you that you missed the island's biggest attraction: the people and their uncanny health. On Crete a heart attack is something exotic. Hardly anyone has one. I think the same could be true in Britain or the U.S. Because the big secret in Crete is no secret at all. A healthy diet and a healthy lifestyle are the only ingredients of this miracle.

I know this because I have been able to verify it personally. Hardly anyone knows that I travel round the world not on a South African passport, but on a Greek one. It happened like this: in the course of my work as a doctor I treated many Greeks, some of them well known. A few years ago my reputation somehow reached the Greek parliament and it got to the point where a few of its members wanted to confer honorary citizenship on me. I was particularly glad that they decided upon this unanimously. As a result I have been a citizen of Greece for five years now.

Not known to many: I hold Greek citizenship.

But back to Crete. Try to remember what kind of meals you had on your last holiday there. In the evening you went with your family or friends to a nice taverna and ordered one of those wonderful fish delicacies. Yes, one of those with all the vegetables – all fresh. During the meal you drank two or three glasses of red wine. And afterwards you felt great.

Why don't you do this at home as well? The secret is called the Crete Method. It actually has nothing in common with conventional dieting schemes, because there is not a trace of avoiding or sacrificing anything. You get whatever is to be had from the kitchen and cellar. But there are a few small, yet essential differences: virtually everything that lands in the pot there comes from the region itself and is, of course, fresh.

Olive oil has for generations had a cult following. Meat is eaten seldom, vegetables much more often, and naturally there is always red wine on the table. Meals are served in a very relaxed atmosphere.

Vegetables, oil, and red wine keep people healthy? Obviously:

- Heart and circulatory disease are virtually unknown in Crete. A comparative study found that heart problems occur 95% less often than in the United States or Europe.
- A test check-up done by the American Society for Prevention found that patients with heart problems who changed their diets to the Crete Method were able to reduce their heart attack risk by 70%.
- Astoundingly, the positive effects of the Crete Method were clearly measurable within six weeks of the dietary change.

The amazing thing about Greek cuisine is not that it is so healthy but that its power could have remained undiscovered for so long. While the whole world was concerning itself with cholesterol and fatty acids, the islanders of Crete were taking a daily dose of olive oil. According to contemporary wisdom, they should promptly have fallen over and died. However, exactly the opposite happened. People who had their daily amount of olive oil were particularly lively and lived to a ripe old age.

This paradox did not remain hidden to all experts. The American researcher Ancel Keys (coincidentally working in Minnesota at the same hospital as I was at the time) was the first to compare the death rate charts relating to heart and circulatory disease of seven countries. His findings showed that such diseases are virtually unknown in Crete. Keys originally published his findings in 1970, but amazingly his results found little resonance. Only when the results were published again in the early 1990s did his findings put Crete soundly on the health map.

Yet it had been known for years that the diet of the peoples in southern European countries could prevent heart diseases. The evidence was provided by one of the largest research studies ever undertaken: MONICA. No, this does not refer to a woman but to a study by dozens of scientists commissioned by the World Health Organization (WHO). The goal was to establish a means of comparing death rates from individual countries according to cause. MONICA lasted for a period of 15 years and included 41 cities in many different countries. When the study was finished in 1995 one could see where heart diseases were most common and where they were not.

World Heart Champions

MONICA completely changed the accepted way of thinking concerning the connection between diet and heart diseases. All of a sudden it became apparent that the healthiest people were those whom nutritionists feared like the devil fears holy water. People for whom food is a lifestyle: the French.

The French emerged as world champions of the healthy heart. This despite the fact that they smoke more, drink more alcohol, and do less exercise than the rest of the world's population.

Explanations for this "French paradox" followed quickly and plentifully. They eat more fruit and vegetables, use high-quality oils, drink red wine, and have an all-round healthier lifestyle. This combination of factors was thought to be the explanation why the inhabitants of Strasbourg had a three times lower risk of dying from a heart attack than the residents of Glasgow.

> *Heart diseases are 10 times less prevalent on Crete than in the rest of Europe.*

But then came Crete. All of a sudden all nutrition researchers had a new passion. As studies showed, this island in the Aegean had a 10 times lower ratio of heart diseases than the rest of Europe. And its cancer death rate was 50% less than in Italy. All of a sudden the health of the French no longer appeared as sensational as before. The whole world was intent on researching the miracle of Crete.

Today we know that this miracle stands on 10 legs:

1 Fruit and vegetables are the main ingredients of the diet.
2 The consumption of meat is 32% and that of sausages 54% less than in northern Europe.
3 Vegetables are cooked with care. Therefore less of the valuable substances they contain, such as vitamins, are lost.
4 Only high-quality fat is used (mostly olive oil).
5 On Crete, 18% more fish is eaten than in northern Europe.
6 The dishes are well seasoned, mostly with strong herbs.
7 Main courses are seldom lavish. Dessert usually consists of fruit or cheese.
8 Red wine is part of the lifestyle and drunk regularly.
9 There are few meals, but these are extended ones.
10 The lifestyle in Crete has little stress. There are plenty of times for relaxing (midday, Sundays).

> *The 10 secrets of the Crete kitchen: a lot of fruit, vegetables, fish, and a stress-free lifestyle.*

I can only recommend: take Crete home – I'm certain you can find a way to integrate a great deal of the diet and some of the lifestyle into your everyday life. Of course you have less time for this in your normal working life than during your holidays. But many of the dishes from the Crete kitchen are so simple that they could almost be called "fast food." More good news: since people living in Mediterranean countries – despite their high consumption of olive oil – generally eat 50% less fat than the residents of northern Europe, you could even lose a few pounds with the Crete diet. This is the first time that fast food could lead to weight loss.

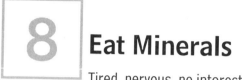

8 Eat Minerals

Tired, nervous, no interest in sex?

Perhaps you're missing important minerals.

Magic Magnesium

Boy, how easy everything seems today. You've never beaten the guy on the other side of the net before. Actually he plays tennis much better than you do, but today it's a different story. You won the first set 6–3, and are now 5–2 up in the second, serving at 40–15. You need only one more point and victory is yours.

Your opponent cracks a mighty serve into your side of the court, but what difference does that make today? You respond with a forehand that you could kiss your hands for. Your opponent can just barely get to the ball and hit it back. It drops very softly over the net and will land somewhere to the right on your side of the court. No problem, that's an easy shot. Two steps and you reach the ball. One. And then: all of a sudden your lower leg no longer follows your command and cramps up. From one second to the next you can't manage another step. The ball bounces once, then twice and a third time. That doesn't interest you at the moment. You just manage to drag yourself to a chair at the side of the court and are trying to massage your leg back into shape. You can finish the game, but the victory that was so close you could smell it is no longer within reach.

> *Too little magnesium will make you a loser at sport – and in the office.*

Later, a club colleague who has seen the match comes up to you and says: "You should take magnesium, old boy. You will see that cramp will be a thing of the past." And it's true. You play your next match without any problems. There's no sign of cramp. It doesn't matter that you lose again.

Zinc for Better Sex

A so-called "light mineral deficit" is more common than people think. You feel listless, tired, and without energy. Your performance in sport is drastically impaired. You are worn out, nervous, and have trouble concentrating. You don't have much of an appetite and have difficulty sleeping. At the office you're always the first to catch a cold and the last to get rid of it.

> *A bad diet and the wrong way of cooking are the main causes of mineral deficiency.*

For many years minerals were not considered very important. Now an increasing amount of evidence is being uncovered showing just what incredible assistance minerals can offer the body. Magnesium to combat stress, selenium for the heart, zinc for colds, calcium for osteoporosis, and zinc again for an increased sex drive. The healthful possibilities are ever increasing.

We can rarely meet all the requirements our daily routine demands of us.

- We eat an improper diet. It is not properly balanced. We don't eat enough vegetables and fruit.
- We do not cook properly. We cook our meals so long that many valuable vitamins and minerals are practically cooked away.
- We don't live correctly. We create too much stress at our job as well as in our free time. Therefore we use up more minerals than before.

- We think incorrectly. We are increasingly fooled by food products that only give the impression of containing large amounts of minerals. But the bright green spinach has 68% less magnesium content than 15 years ago. Carrots have lost 57% of their magnesium content, potatoes a third and broccoli has a quarter less. Just a few years ago a basket of vegetables contained 30% more magnesium than it does today.

> *Mineral deficiency is more common today than vitamin deficiency.*

Our food products have not been cast under a spell that's made them lose their minerals. A vicious circle of misdeeds is to blame, first in the soil, then in the plants, and then in animals and humans. Magnesium is just one mineral washed out of the earth by acid rain.

Too Little Selenium and Calcium

Where do we have our greatest deficiencies? In the case of magnesium, a German study has found evidence that the right amount can only be maintained with great difficulty through our normal diet. A study in Vienna and environs found that three-quarters of all people examined had a zinc and/or a selenium deficiency. According to a German nutrition report, one in every three children, one in four young adults, and one in five women suffer from a calcium deficiency. The results of a study by the Institute for Sports Medicine in Freiburg showed that one in five athletes has disturbingly low potassium levels. The consequence of this, besides a lapse in achievement levels, is reduced heart performance.

Minerals are absolutely essential for our bodies. Without them our organism could not function. Muscles, brain, nerves, and heart would be missing the fuel they need to function.

MINERAL GUIDE
The Most Important Minerals and Trace Elements

Mineral	Main Importance	Main Sources
Magnesium	heart, nerves, blood	grain, vegetables, nuts
Sodium	muscles, nerves, water balance	drinking water, salt
Calcium	heart, muscles, nerves, bones	cocoa, vegetables, parsley
Potassium	blood, bones, teeth	milk, nuts, vegetables
Iron	blood, muscles, breathing	peas, beans, grains
Fluoride	bones, teeth	fish, black tea, walnuts
Iodine	metabolism, thyroid gland	fish, seafood, spinach
Selenium	cells, immune system, heart	rice, offal, grain
Silicon	bones, skin, hair	potatoes, mineral water
Zinc	growth, sexual hormones	rolled oats, offal, cheese

The most important minerals and trace elements for our heart: potassium, magnesium, and selenium.

Magnesium is practically the oil for the heart motor. Without magnesium the so-called ionic pumps of the heart are not capable of ensuring the regulated process of the systoles and the diastoles. Potassium, on the other hand, is the fuel for the motor. If the oil pumps are not working properly, the fuel supply does not function well either. It doesn't seem logical to me to take good care of the pump but neglect the fuel supply.

There are many studies which confirm the positive effects of magnesium on the heart. The most spectacular of these was the British LIMIT study undertaken in 1992. Patients who were suspected of having had a heart attack were given a magnesium injection. This reduced the death rate by 25%.

Other impressive evidence of just how greatly magnesium can raise performance capabilities was discovered by Austrian researchers in combination with experts from the United States Air Force Academy in Colorado Springs. Soldiers were given strenuous physical tasks to do. After one week, the group given magnesium capsules beforehand was able to achieve 30% more than the other.

Potassium Against High Blood Pressure

Potassium plays a major role in the battle against high blood pressure, one of the biggest risk factors for heart attacks. In the industrial countries, one in five people suffers from high blood pressure. In Germany alone the number is 10 million. In the over-65 age group, one in two suffers from hypertension.

High blood pressure reduces life expectancy drastically. Studies have shown that a 45-year-old man with normal blood pressure levels has an average of 32 more years left to live. A man the same age with high blood pressure has on average only 20.5 years left to live. The guidelines today are: the systolic blood pressure level should not be higher than 140 mm/Hg, the diastolic reading should not be higher than 90 mm/Hg. According to the World Health Organization, the old guidelines (100 + one's plus age) are no longer relevant.

Also no longer relevant is the opinion that salt alone is the decisive factor in the development of hypertension. In the meantime it has become known that one in two cases of high blood pressure has a genetic cause. A research study at the University of Bonn also found evidence that a stringent low-salt diet has much less effect than previously thought. Only one in three patients in the study was able to lower his blood pressure through dietary measures alone. In 16% of patients, blood pressure levels actually rose. This shows that salt alone is not the cause of hypertension. The key is the relationship between sodium and potassium. A lot of sodium and very little potassium – blood pressure shoots up.

Don't pave the way for a heart attack. Eat your minerals!

9 No Cholesterol Stress, Please

It can be useful to know your cholesterol level.
However, there are more important things in life.

I n the U.S., cholesterol is as well known as Coca-Cola and McDonald's. In no other country in the world do so many people know something about their blood fat levels. Nowhere else do people take so much medication to reduce their cholesterol levels – namely nine million units per year. In no other country is the turnover of low cholesterol or cholesterol-free food products so high. The battle against fat has taken on the dimensions of a crusade in America.

A study by the U.S. National Heart, Lung, and Blood Institute revealed the following:

- 75% of all Americans have had at least one cholesterol test. This is 10% more than nine years ago and double that of 1983.

Every second American can inform you about his cholesterol level at any time.

- 49% can spontaneously give you their cholesterol readings – 16 times more than in 1983.
- One in five Americans was told by his doctor that his cholesterol readings were too high.

50

- Currently, 69% know that a cholesterol level under 200 serves as a guideline base.

In a country that has even initiated a national cholesterol education program, a recent report naturally caused a major uproar: America's largest medical specialists' organization, the American College of Physicians, representing 85,000 internists in the U.S., called for a drastic reduction in cholesterol tests. As recently as 1998 they had recommended screenings for everyone between the ages of 20 and 70. Now the experts have done an about-face and recommend:

- No more cholesterol tests for men under the age of 35.
- No more cholesterol tests for women under the age of 45.
- No more cholesterol tests for people over the age of 75.

For the age groups in between, cholesterol tests are appropriate but by no means necessary. It cannot be conclusively derived from the latest study if screenings are necessary in the above-65 age group. Naturally, these guidelines only have validity when no definitive risk factors such as high blood pressure, diabetes, or a family history of heart problems are present.

The reason for this radical re-evaluation by the specialists is quite astounding as well. Apparently there is no evidence that a low cholesterol level in younger people has any bearing on the heart attack risk. In the case of older people there is absolutely no relevant study concerning cholesterol as a factor for heart and circulatory problems. Dr. Alan Garber, professor at the University of Stanford and one of the authors of the new guidelines, had the following to say about the new developments: "Our reservations come from the fact that we prescribe medication for younger people – and this for years – without knowing that they actually provide any advantages."

> For years cholesterol was the villain. Now it has been given absolution.

So what is happening here? For years cholesterol was the villain and now all of a sudden it receives doctors' blessing. Is cholesterol no longer an enemy of the heart? Can we eat according to our heart's desire without regret? No, because cholesterol remains a risk factor for heart and circulatory diseases. Whether it truly plays the major role, as was assumed for so many years, will only be revealed over the course of the next years by research studies.

Good Cholesterol

Cholesterol is a waxy, fatty substance. Don't confuse it with a poison, because you can't live without cholesterol. It is important for cells, nerves, and hormones. Our liver uses it in order to make bile. Eighty percent of the body's cholesterol is produced in the liver; only 20% is absorbed through our diet.

Fat cannot be dissolved by the blood and therefore cannot be transported. For this cholesterol needs a coat of proteins, so-called aproteins. As a duo they appear under the name of lipoproteins.

There are various types of lipoproteins. Two types that you should be acquainted with:

- LDL (low-density) cholesterol, also known as "bad cholesterol"
- HDL (high-density) cholesterol, also known as "good cholesterol."

The differentiation between good and bad has a solid basis. If there is too much LDL cholesterol in the blood, the excess is oxidized and deposited on the inside walls of the arteries. This is the moment HDL cholesterol has been waiting for. Its job is to "grab" the excess LDL cholesterol and transport it to the liver for disposal. If the balance between LDL and HDL cholesterol is disturbed, then LDL particles are stored on the inside of the arteries. This leads to narrowing of the arteries, termed arteriosclerosis, which can cause heart disease or even a heart attack.

More and more experts are saying that healthy people should simply ignore their cholesterol level if it is below 300 mg/dl.

In order to find out if your cholesterol is balanced you have to take a test. This test checks your overall cholesterol level, your HDL readings, your LDL level, and your level of triglycerides (another fat compound). The blood levels are measured in milligrams per deciliter (mg/dl).

Cholesterol Levels for a Healthy Adult (mg/dl)

Blood Fat	Desired	Borderline	Undesirable
Total Cholesterol	under 200	200 – 240	over 240
LDL	under 130	130 – 160	over 160
Triglycerides	under 200	200 – 400	over 400
HDL	over 45	35 – 45	under 35

These guideline levels are coming under increasing criticism, however. Studies have shown that a blood fat reading of under 300 mg/dl creates no measurable heart attack risk. One of the best-known experts, Professor Hans-Jürgen Holtmeier of the University of Freiburg (Germany) states: "Healthy people should not be bothered by cholesterol levels under 300 mg/dl."

The confusion over cholesterol began some 30 years ago and is chronicled by overambitious research mixed with many contradictions.

- The discovery phase. In the 1960s research showed that people with high cholesterol were more prone to heart disease. Theory: cholesterol is deposited on the inner walls of the arteries, thereby hindering blood flow.

Eggs used to be thought of as cholesterol monsters. Now they are recommended.

- The recommendation phase. After the first phase, a series of recommendations was published with information on how to keep one's cholesterol level in check. Plant-derived margarines instead of butter, fewer eggs, and very little meat were recommended.

- The surprise phase. Medical experts then discovered that cholesterol levels in the body could not be regulated so easily. With some people, the level remained the same regardless of what they ate. With others, who tried all sorts of difficult diets, it still wouldn't go down. Many who suffered a heart attack had low cholesterol.

- The easing phase. Experts began to look at cholesterol from different perspectives. The total cholesterol level was no longer of relevance, but the individual levels for HDL and LDL cholesterol as well as for triglycerides were now considered important. As a result of the new findings, recommendations for a "correct cholesterol diet" were revised as well. Eggs were removed from the forbidden list, because even though they contain high levels of cholesterol they also contain a great deal of unsaturated fat, considered very healthy. The recommendations for red meat (eat in moderation) and butter (use sparingly) remained intact. Additions to the recommended list were foods used in Mediterranean cuisine such as fish and olive oil.

Margarine: recommended at first, now put on the blacklist.

Then came the next shock. The much praised alternative to butter, plant-derived margarine, was found to be a virtual cholesterol minefield. Findings showed that in the hardening process of the natural oil, trans-fatty acids are created which raise the LDL (bad cholesterol) and triglycerides to alarming levels. The situation was a paradox. Of all substances it was fat-free margarine which had been sent into the front line of the battle against cholesterol; now it had proved to be a treacherous cholesterol enhancer.

But that was not all. Besides HDL, LDL, and triglycerides, a new form of fat appeared: lipoprotein (a) or Lp(a), also called "bad cholesterol II" because it possesses the same characteristics as LDL cholesterol. The difference is that Lp(a) cannot be controlled by a change in eating habits, as LDL can, because Lp(a) is largely genetically determined. Anyone with a high Lp(a) level can only try to keep other risk factors for heart disease down to a minimum.

Now you're probably thinking, "what should I do after all these contradictory studies and opinions?" Don't do anything. It really doesn't make any difference if cholesterol is very bad or only a little bad. A person eating a healthy diet should do it for the sake of their whole body, not to attain the correct cholesterol level. A balanced diet has many positive effects. If along the way you manage to lower your cholesterol, well that's wonderful. If you're not able to do this, you are nevertheless getting what you need in vitamins, minerals, trace elements, and other nutrients. This will help extend your life.

Barnard Tips for a Healthy Heart

Ten Ways to Keep Cholesterol in Check

1 **Be realistic.**
   Accept the fact that a high cholesterol level increases the chances of a heart attack.

2 **Keep your perspective.**
   Being overweight, smoking, and high blood pressure are often more dangerous than cholesterol.

3 **React correctly.**
   Whatever the truth about cholesterol, you should still eat a healthy diet.

4 **Be skeptical.**
   Not everything that says "low cholesterol" actually is.

5 **Live naturally.**
   Eat fresh produce from your region as often as you can. You're usually on the safe side if you do.

6 **Keep your feet firmly on the ground.**
   Flexibility is good, but meat and animal fats should not be your main source of nourishment.

7 **Be choosy.**
   A good olive oil should be as important to you as a good bottle of wine.

8 **Use nature's arsenal.**
   Garlic and avocados are nature's weapons against too much cholesterol.

9 **Don't lie to yourself.**

Fish is good in the battle against cholesterol, but deep-fried battered cod is not what we're talking about here.

10 **Exercise.**

Three times a week for 30 minutes brings your cholesterol levels back down to earth.

10 Live Naturally

You probably know that fruit and vegetables are good for you. But did you know that the same applies to nuts and chocolate?

Where will our food come from in the year 2010? From the laboratory? From nature? Or perhaps it will be a combination of the two. Believe me: you will be confronted by this question much more often and urgently than you might think now.

What has happened up to now: nature is not perfect, that we're aware of. Fruits and vegetables do not grow throughout the year, generally spoil quickly, and can often look pretty awful. Grain used to taste bitter, butter could not be taken fresh out of the refrigerator and spread on a piece of bread. So man decided to doctor around a bit with nature. Fruit and vegetables are now harvested before they ripen and then synthetically ripened. The bitter substances were cultivated out of grain. Butter was made "spreadable" with the addition of other substances.

So everything's OK? Absolutely not, for people are ungrateful. They find synthetically ripened fruit tasteless, search increasingly for natural breads, and want their proper butter back. For the food industry it means back to the drawing board to come up with something new. So what is new? Well, nothing is being added to fruit and vegetables, instead, something's being taken out – those active substances that we know are good for humans. Pills or powders are then made from them. It seems like a logical idea. In the morning you drink coffee and take a pill and, hey presto, you have given yourself the most important plant substances needed for the day.

> *Nutrition's big leap into the future: food and active plant substances unite.*

But it can be done even more cleverly. The coffee you buy can already contain the necessary active plant substances. You don't need any more pills. Visions of the future? No, because in the United States something like this is already available, called either "functional food," "medical food," or "nutraceuticals." If you speak to a corporate executive from a food corporation about this, his eyes will light up because this may yet prove to be the nutrition industry's big business idea. For about a year now, a company known for its soups, has been offering 40 packaged meals, from breakfast to dinner – with home delivery. Blood pressure can be reduced through a combination of active plant substances in these products, cholesterol can be lowered, and help provided in combating diabetes. According to *Newsweek*, eight university studies can confirm the effect of these products.

> *Plants contain 10,000 different substances which can help prevent cancer and heart disease.*

"Functional food" probably has its positive aspects. Maybe in a few years we will be able to combat heart disease and cancer with hamburgers and french fries. But we shouldn't exaggerate the power of the lab. The best weapons against disease can still be found in nature. Fruit and vegetables don't only contain one substance, but a whole array of active substances that can help combat heart disease and prevent cancer. At least 10,000 different substances, perhaps even more, are said to be contained in our plants. We only know of the positive effects of a few; experts say this is only the beginning.

The Wonder of Nature

The food industry has a very mighty opponent. Let's take a closer look at it. Plants look pretty simple, however on the inside they're little miracles, much too complicated to have been made by man. They are fuelled by the so-called secondary active plant substances or bio-active substances.

> *When you eat fruit and vegetables, you are also swallowing the "defence army" contained in these natural foods.*

It's with these active substances that plants ward off enemies, attract beneficial insects, regulate growth and water balance, as well as control their coloring. These secondary substances are becoming increasingly important to mankind, because every time you eat fruit, vegetables, or herbs you are eating the complete package. And they have an amazing effect, because bio-active substances can:

- help to lower the risk of cancer
- be good for the heart, because they inhibit the production of free radicals and can lower cholesterol levels
- strengthen the immune system
- protect against infections from fungi, viruses, and bacteria.

The good thing about this is that you can taste it. Pick a ripe tomato from the garden and bite into it. You probably will think it is a different kind of vegetable than the bright red ones you buy at the supermarket.

Nature has even more to offer: herbs. For hundreds of years herbs have been used effectively in the battle against disease, and many have found their way into medicines. One need only think of digitalis, the active substance found in the purple foxglove, which for 200 years has been used around the world as a heart stimulant.

Natural remedies are increasing in popularity around the world. Americans currently spend $12 billion a year on natural remedies, double the amount spent only five years ago. In Germany it's 10 billion marks. Almost 60 million Americans take medication based on active plant substances. While the discussion of the pharmaceutical wonder drug "Prozac" is raging around the world, 7.7 million Americans are already taking its plant-based counterpart:

an extract from a yellow flower called St John's wort. Another extract, ginkgo biloba (taken from the bark of a tree) is said to help protect against memory loss and help battle impotence. According to a report in *Newsweek*, 10.8 million Americans are already converts.

The cornucopia of active substances contained in plants can hardly be cataloged. From the rain forests of the Amazon to the Black Forest, new substances are constantly being discovered that give hope of protection against, a treatment or a cure for, various diseases. The German Society for Nutrition has compiled a list of the most important active secondary plant substances:

- Carotenoids (pigments). The most important are betacarotene, found in yellow- and orange-coloured fruit and vegetables such as apricots and carrots, and xanthophyll, found in green-leafed vegetables such as spinach and cabbage. Carotenoids are good for the heart, support the immune system, and fight cancer.
- Phytosterol. This can be found mostly in plant seeds and in plant oils. It helps to reduce cholesterol levels in the blood.
- Saponins. Bitter substances found in peas and beans. They lower cholesterol and fight cancer.
- Glucosinolate. They're responsible for the typical taste of mustard, horse radish, and kohlrabi. They fight free radicals and protect against infections.
- Polyphenoles. Phenol acids and flavonoids are examples of these, found largely in the outer skins of fruit, vegetables and wholemeal grains. They are effective against cancer, battle infection, and protect the heart from oxidizing radicals.

Chocolate contains 20 times as many polyphenoles as the highly recommended tomato does.

- Protease inhibitors. These are enzymes that inhibit the reduction of plant proteins. They can be found in peas and beans. They have an antioxidant effect and reduce blood sugar levels.
- Monoterpenes. These are effective against cancer. They can be found in peppermint and citrus oils.

- Phyto-oestrogens can be found in soya beans, wholemeal products, and linseed. They combat cancer and free radicals.
- Sulfides. The most important representative is garlic with the active substance alliin, which lowers blood pressure and can have an antioxidant effect.
- Lectin. Can be found in peas and beans as well as grain products, and can lower the blood sugar levels.

10 HERBS AND SPICES THAT ARE GOOD FOR THE HEART

	Effects
Whitethorn	Increases blood flow in the heart. Effective against feelings of pressure on the heart.

> *Nature's weapons against heart disease: whitethorn, rose hip, Allium ursinum.*

Allium ursinum	The leaves are filled with vitamin C. Protects against arteriosclerosis.
Elderberry	The berries contain a large amount of vitamin C and minerals. The blossoms strengthen the immune system.
Lavender	Increases blood flow, effective against stress, strengthens nerves, and helps with sleeplessness.
Balm	Soothes and helps you to sleep well. Effective against digestive problems.
Valerian	Reduces stress, is good for the nerves and a good night's sleep.
Rose hip	Contains a large amount of vitamin C. Seven grams are enough for the average daily requirement.
Sea buckthorn	Contains vitamin E, B-complex, minerals. The berries are filled with vitamin C.
Cinnamon	Effective against flatulence, which can cause pressure on the heart, as well as providing relief for bloating.
Yarrow	Contains many bitter substances, acts as an antiseptic, and helps the digestive process.

10 FRUITS AND VEGETABLES THAT ARE GOOD FOR THE HEART

	Effects
Tomatoes	Have the most vitamin E of all plants. Can combat arteriosclerosis.

> *Grapefruit contains substances which can reduce cholesterol.*

Red peppers	Have more vitamin C than kiwi fruit. A good source of betacarotene.
Spinach	Has less iron than once thought, but a good source of betacarotene.
Grapefruit	Has a great amount of vitamin C and betacarotene. Contains substances that can lower cholesterol.
Carrots	Also a good source of betacarotene. One hundred grams suffice for the daily requirement.
Broccoli	Contains a great amount of vitamin C. Sixty grams provide the daily requirement. Also contains calcium and iron.
Onion	Jack of all trades in the body. Lowers blood pressure. Supports the good cholesterol.
Garlic	Vitamins A, C and E. Also contains selenium. Reduces cholesterol and strengthens the immune system.
Strawberries	Have more vitamin C than lemons. Protect the cells. Combat oxidation.
Avocado	Contains a great amount of unsaturated fatty acids, vitamin D, and potassium. An ally against cholesterol.

The research into secondary plant substances is suddenly giving new life to foods which for years were on the "to avoid at all costs" list – chocolate, for instance. This sugar-filled delicacy was condemned for years, but is now considered practically medicinal. Researchers at the University of Scranton in Pennsylvania discovered that chocolate is good for the heart and the immune system. It contains polyphenoles which battle free radicals and help lower cholesterol. Chocolate contains 20 times more polyphenoles than the much-praised tomato and double the amount found in garlic.

The higher the amount of cocoa in a chocolate product, the more valuable the substances it contains.

Nuts were also not looked upon too kindly in years past. From a nutritional standpoint they were considered useless; it was said all they did was make you fat. Now new findings have revealed that they are rich in vitamins and minerals. An American study also found that they contain a great deal of unsaturated fatty acids, which can help lower cholesterol. A second American study also proved that nuts can have a protective effect on the heart. Nurses in Boston who ate 150 grams of nuts a week had a heart attack risk that was one-third below average.

The research into the wonders of nature is only just beginning. Nutritional specialist Dr. Ronald Krauss of the Lawrence Berkley Laboratory said recently in *Time* magazine: "It is much too early to steer the research results in any particular direction, all we can currently say is: eat more fruit and vegetables."

Stress

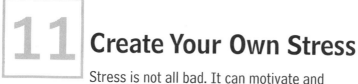

11 | Create Your Own Stress

Stress is not all bad. It can motivate and create self-confidence. The body's true enemy is constant haste.

Sophia Loren was once visiting New York when burglars broke into her hotel suite. They demanded all her jewellery and threatened to kill her children if she did not comply. She had no choice but to open the safe and give them the jewels.

> *"Never cry over things that can't cry over you."* Sophia Loren

Sophia told me this disturbing story a little while after it had occurred. I offered my sympathy and said that I could understand that she was sad about the loss of her jewellery. She only shrugged her shoulders and said: "You know, I have a motto in life, never to cry over things that cannot cry over you."

This statement impressed me immensely because there is a great deal of wisdom behind it. Many things which upset us and worry us constantly are simply not worth it. Over the span of my career my experiences have shown me that 90% of all situations that cause us stress turn out to be trivial and inconsequential.

I have always had a rather relaxed approach towards stress. I never saw it as something innately bad. Stress can be immensely motivating – it can challenge us. It forces us to confront a situation emotionally.

I don't think I would have become a good doctor without a certain amount of stress. I always wanted to be there 100% for my patients. If someone was ill in my clinic, I could think of nothing else all day. The pressure I was under allowed me to care even more intensively for my patients. I wanted to know everything about their illness. Therefore stress was, in my job, a kind of engine that drove me to do better and more.

The problem with stress today is that this engine no longer listens. Strangely enough there are more and more discoveries that supposedly make our jobs and life easier, but never before have so many people complained about being overwhelmed.

> *Every third person suffers from too much stress at work.*

- Stress is becoming more common: one in three suffers from too much pressure at work.
- Stress is getting younger: half of 31- to 45-year-olds feel overwhelmed at work.
- Stress is affecting more women. Currently 40% of women feel overworked either at work or at home. The double role of working mother is an increasing burden for women. Half feel that they are subjected to increased stress.
- Stress is becoming more and more dangerous: in the United States, 60% of all work-related accidents are the direct result of overwork.

Stress now occurs in all professions and at all social levels. It used to be known as the curse of managers, but that was long ago. An investigation by the World Health Organization revealed that workers and other employed people are more stress-prone than the self-employed. The less a person is allowed to make his or her own decisions, the more likely he or she is to feel overburdened.

Valium against Stress

We don't show much imagination in the things we do to combat stress. Many merely take a sedative. I think that these drugs are taken too lightly. This method also only treats the symptom, not the cause.

I used to know a pharmacist in a small town in South Africa. He was very popular in his town because no matter what little problem someone had, he always knew of some way to treat it. One day he had to go away for a while and his assistant took over. During his absence a patient entered the pharmacy and complained of severe diarrhea. The assistant looked around among the bottles of medicine but did not have a clue what to suggest. Eventually his eyes fell on a bottle of Valium. He said to himself, "Maybe if I calm the patient down, the diarrhea will also stop." When the pharmacist eventually returned and heard what the assistant had done, he was horrified and immediately dismissed him. A few days later the poor assistant, now jobless, was wandering the streets when he met the man he'd sold the Valium to. He thought to himself, "I'll ask him whether it was any help." So he walked up and said, "Excuse me, sir, do you remember me?" "Yes – You gave me the medicine for my diarrhea." The assistant asked him, "Tell me, sir, did the medicine help?" The man thought for a bit and then replied: "To tell you the truth, it *did* help. I still soil my pants, but I don't worry about it anymore."

Stress is in fashion. We use it as a reference for anything we find negative in our lives. But who decides if we are challenged by a situation or put under pressure by it? We do. Put yourself in the following situation. Five minutes before it's quitting time, your boss comes over to you to say she wants a three-page speech typed out by the next morning. This puts you under pressure because you have theater tickets for the evening. What do you do? You quickly type up the speech, race home to change, and then rush to the theater. You arrive five minutes before the performance starts. In the foyer you have a quick smoke and then fall, exhausted, into your seat. You experience stress negatively, blaming it for your exhaustion and inability to follow what's happening on stage. In fact, you blame everyone and everything but yourself.

Who really decides whether you will suffer from stress or not? You do!

You could have looked upon this situation as a challenge. You could have decided to come in half an hour early next day and type it up. This would have allowed you to have a wonderful evening at the theater and you wouldn't have had any stress. What I would like to point out with this example is the following:

- You alone decide – most of the time – if you are subjected to stress or not.
- Much that we call stress is really impatience and haste. These are your body's real enemies.

Looking at it this way makes it seem relatively easy to deal with stress, at least initially. Think about what has caused you tension over the course of the last few days; probably a few trivial things which by now seem silly to have got upset about.

STRESS CHECK: HOW HIGH IS YOUR STRESS FACTOR?

The American stress researcher Steve Burns has developed a scale with which to measure stress levels. Make a note of every occurrence that you have experienced over the past 12 months, and of its stress factor.

1 Death of a partner/loved one	100
2 Divorce	60
3 Mid-life crisis	60

Anything can cause stress: an argument with your boss, problems with your sex life, or a parking ticket.

4 Separation from a partner/loved one	60
5 Prison or suspended sentence	60
6 Death of family member	60
7 Severe injury or illness	45
8 Marriage	45
9 Getting fired/losing a job	45
10 Reconciliation with a partner/lover	40
11 Retirement	40

12	Serious illness of a family member	40
13	Job with more than a 40-hour week	35
14	Pregnancy of a partner/lover	35
15	Problems in one's sex life	35
16	New family member	35
17	A change in profession or status	35
18	Change in financial status	35
19	Death of a close friend	30
20	Altercations with a partner/lover	25
21	Mortgage, credit, loan	25
22	Premature settlement of loan, credit	25
23	Less than 8 hours' sleep at night	25
24	Change of responsibilities at work	25
25	Problems with your children	25
26	Extraordinary physical performance (exertion)	25
27	Partner starts to work or retires	20
28	Starting or finishing school	20
29	Change in living environment (renovation, new cleaning lady, guests, etc.)	20
30	Change in daily habits (diet, fitness training, quitting smoking)	20
31	Chronic allergies	20
32	Problems with one's superiors (boss)	20
33	Change in work habits or conditions	15
34	Move to a new house, apartment	15
35	The days leading up to a woman's monthly period	15
36	Changes at school	15
37	Change in religious activities	15
38	Change in social activities	15
39	A pay cut	10
40	Change in the frequency of family gatherings	10
41	Holiday	10
42	Wintertime	10
43	Minor infraction of the law (e.g., parking ticket)	5

Now add up your score.

Red Zone: More than 250 points. Your stress factor has reached a dangerous level.

Yellow Zone: More than 150 points. You can only cope with your stress if you learn to deal with it correctly.

Green Zone: Fewer than 150 points. Life is good to you.

Stress is not the enemy we have tended to take it for; in truth it is our ally. It serves us as the perfect alibi for our bad habits. Just listen to people give their reasons for smoking, drinking, eating too quickly or too much (or too little!), not exercising, and not having any time for their family. Correct: because they feel stressed.

In my life I've been under stress only three times that I think worth talking about. All three times had to do with people who were very close to me. When my second wife, Barbara, divorced me it was a new and painful experience for me: separation from a person can sometimes cause more stress than their death. When my father died it caused me a great deal of grief. He was a very charismatic man and we were very close. He died suddenly.

My third major stress experience came when my eldest son and I were on holiday together. He was 10 at the time. He woke up suddenly one night gasping for breath. I thought he had croup and realized that he might need a tracheotomy, but I had no surgery instruments available. I gave him some of the medicine I had available and put him in the bathroom, which I filled with steam by turning on a hot shower. Suddenly he vomited and, like magic, the obstruction in his air passage disappeared. When I was back in Cape Town I consulted a pediatrician, who informed me that my son had suffered from a laryngeal spasm which disappears after a bout of vomiting.

Stress Motivates

With this example I have tried to depict a further good side to stress. It puts our bodies in the optimal position to react properly to the outside world. In former times this tension prepared us for a battle or for flight. In our modern world, stress ensures that we are prepared to cope with the challenges we encounter in our jobs and in our private lives. In my case stress helped me overcome sadness, death, and potential danger.

> *Most things that cause us stress are not worth it.*

We now know the most important characteristics of stress:

- We are the cause of most stress.
- Most things that cause stress are not worth it.
- Stress is an angel because it motivates and challenges us.
- Stress is a devil because it causes us to use it as an excuse.

The pioneer of stress research, Hans Selye, divided stress into two sub-categories: *distress* and *eustress.*

Eustress describes positive pressure: situations which give us pleasant feelings such as the happy anticipation of a rendezvous, a marriage, a pay rise, starting a new chapter in our lives, etc.

Distress is the opposite: we feel distressed when we are faced with a challenge we cannot surmount.

The body initially doesn't differentiate between good and bad stress. The autonomous nerve system automatically initiates the reactions. Hormones are produced, the blood pressure rises, and heart rate increases. The breathing comes faster.

> *The "Schwarzenegger phenomenon": sportsmen and women are better able to cope with stress.*

For the heart, the creation of catecholamines (the stress hormones noradrenaline and adrenaline) is important. The work of these two hormones can be felt quickly: the heart beats more intensely and perhaps more rapidly.

Dr. Sepp Porta, stress researcher from the University of Graz (Austria), established back in 1989 that catecholamines do not have a direct feedback system. This means that the nerve cells and the adrenal body continue to distribute more and more of these hormones, for as long as the stress-causing situation lasts. This is one of the reasons why continual stress is so bad for the heart.

The best cure: sport. The reduction of the catecholamines takes place in the mitochondria, which can be found in all cells including the muscle cells. A physically fit individual has more muscle cells and therefore more mitochondria. Physically fit individuals can reduce catecholamines faster and thereby reduce stress more rapidly as well. Porta jokingly calls this the "Schwarzenegger phenomenon."

Sophia Loren does not have as many muscles as Arnold Schwarzenegger. Therefore you might think she couldn't reduce stress as quickly as he. But her philosophical approach to life ensures that she doesn't take things too much to heart.

Barnard Tips for a Healthy Heart
The 10 Best Methods to Prevent Stress

1 **Don't take everything to heart.**
   90% of the things we get upset about aren't worth it.

2 **Set your priorities.**
   The most important first, the unimportant into the waste basket.

3 **Don't be a dreamer.**
   Set yourself an attainable goal every day.

4 **Manage your body like a machine.**
   Take care of it. Let off steam every now and then.

5 **Take time from others.**
   Why should you always adhere to the schedule of others?

> *Don't expect to put up a world-record performance every day.*

6 **Think positive.**
   Look on stress as a challenge.

7 **Don't be a perfectionist.**
   Don't have unrealistic expectations for yourself or for anyone else.

8 **Think of yourself as replaceable.**
   Holidays are not only for other people.

9 **Let others work.**
   Learn to delegate. Why should you be the only one getting into a sweat?

10 **Show some emotion.**
   Love, grief, passion, etc. help you to release that pent-up energy and clear your thoughts.

12 Tame Your Mobile Phone

Don't let modern technology get you down.
You are the boss. You give the orders.

Technology is a good servant but a poor master. If you allow yourself to be dominated by modern technology, you put yourself under unnecessary pressure. If you know how to use your computer, mobile, or the Internet properly, they can make life easier for you.

I have never allowed myself to be subjected to so-called "techno-stress," either privately or as a doctor. I belong to another generation. I have a computer at home, but I am not even sure how to turn it on. I have had a mobile for a few weeks but no one ever calls me on it because I haven't given anyone the number. During my years as a practicing physician I was not very interested in technology because I was of the opinion that much of it was unnecessary. It's true that some machines and devices can help with diagnoses, but a good doctor can find out more about his patient with his eyes, hands and a stethoscope – though there's also a place for an EEG!

I am of the opinion that, especially in medicine, the use of technology is greatly exaggerated. In many hospitals doctors and nurses no longer watch over patients but rather leave that to high-tech devices. Machines, however, cannot give love.

Nothing has developed so rapidly over the past years as the electronic devices that now surround us every day. Computers, faxes, answering machines, pagers, mobiles, the Internet, e-mail, etc. On its way into the 21st century, humanity is surrounded by technology. It's a status symbol to be constantly reachable. The borders between the world of work and one's private life are becoming more and more blurred. The work day doesn't begin when you get to work, but starts in the car or on the train or bus when you check your voice mail, make or take a few "urgent" calls, or send a fax or e-mail. And the working day only ends when you finally turn your mobile and/or home computer off at night. However, many leave these on round the clock.

All this is leaving its mark on us. In her book *Damn Technology*, the American psychologist Michelle Well states that half of all leading associates, managers, and office workers in the U.S. describe themselves as stressed by technology. Workers have too little control over technology, too little training, and hardly any reprieve from the continual information and innovation flow.

> *Half of all managers in the United States feel "techno-stressed."*

The term "techno-stress" originally described the problems of people who had trouble coming to terms with their computer. Today it connotes all the stress that can be caused by technology: the anger when you cannot find a TV programme, the fear of being under electronic surveillance, or the fear of losing one's job because of technology.

The frustration of being controlled by technology is more and more frequently turning into aggression. The trade magazine *PC World* recently published the results of a survey of American technology bosses. Eighty-three percent of these top managers had already experienced how computer problems resulted in direct attacks on the PC. One in five bosses had to exchange a keyboard which had been broken after an "anger attack." "Flying computer mice" are becoming more frequent, monitors are being increasingly smashed, and hard drives are getting kicked more and more often. American psychologists have given these symptoms a name: "network rage," comparable to the "road rage" frequently encountered when a motorist stuck in traffic feels helpless and lashes out in anger.

> *Techno-stress and its consequences: computers are smashed, mice fly through the air.*

I recently read that in Japan, special relaxation training is being offered. For about $100, stress-plagued individuals can relieve their tensions by smashing office furniture to bits. Included in the price are the necessary tools, as well as sushi and a beer.

Thus we have evidence of the negative aspects of technology:

- More and more people feel pressurized by technology.
- More and more people feel that they are slowly losing control over technology.
- More and more people feel that they cannot keep pace with the speed of innovation.
- More and more people feel bothered by mobiles.
- With increased frequency, this "techno-stress" turns into aggression.

I am not an enemy of technology. I have seen how computers are helpful to others, and even to me. I know that the Internet and e-mail help make life easier, and how television helps increase our knowledge of the world. Yet at the same time I know of nothing that can cause more stress than mobiles and their clones. Everywhere, technology traps abound. If you know where they are, then you will seldom have trouble with them. If you don't know where they are, you will quickly be caught out.

1. The Information Trap

In Germany, every employee, manager, or civil servant receives on average 177 messages by fax, e-mail, telephone, office memo, mobile, or pager per day. Almost two-thirds of these workers have to put up with these interruptions on average every 10 minutes. Our jobs are becoming more erratic – zigzagging back and forth – because in short intervals we have to adapt to new directives. According to a study done by the U.S. firm of Pitney Bowes, 27% of the people in Germany feel overwhelmed by information. Sixty percent of leading managers declare that they have trouble with the dissemination of messages.

The U.S. Information Society has created its own symptom: "Information Fatigue Syndrome," the excessive addiction to messages. The American media critic Neil Postman poses the question: "Are we drowning in a flood of information just like the Sorcerer's Apprentice?"

2. The Television Trap

Nothing has changed our lives so dramatically over the past decades as television. It has left its mark on what we think about the modern world. Our social contacts have been channelled into new paths and our forms of communication changed.

The German Economic Institute has calculated that adults spend on average 10 years of their lives in front of the television. Germans watch almost $3^{1}/_{2}$ hours of TV a day – almost double the amount they were watching 15 years ago.

American children watch "the boob tube" an average of 17 hours a week. A research study by the University of Stanford revealed that watching television is one of the main causes of obesity in the U.S.A. A control group of 8- to 10-year-olds who, over a span of one year, watched 25% less television gained, on average, two pounds less than other children of the same age group.

> *Television is one of the main causes of obesity in the U.S.A.*

Television not only makes people fat, but it is addictive as well. A five-year study by the British Film Institute found that most of those questioned claimed TV was "trivial garbage," but "could not stop watching it." Many feel "guilty" watching TV, yet find it provides "relief from stress."

3. The Internet Trap

The number of Internet users is exploding around the world. Whether you're in New York or in Timbuktu, you have access to virtually endless information. You can read newspapers, sell your car, book your next holiday, do bank transactions, participate in games of chance, and even have sex on-line.

> *By 2005, a billion people will be surfing the net.*

Two-thirds of Americans currently use the Internet, while one in three Germans has a connection either in the office or at home. Over 300 million people around the world are members of the Internet community. Every 15 months this figure doubles. By the year 2005, a billion people will be surfing the net. The World Wide Web will change our lives as dramatically as television did in the 1950s:

- It will transform us into a total information society.
- It will change the way we work. Many jobs will disappear, others will be created.
- Our leisure time will be restructured.
- It will revolutionize our shopping habits.
- Our sex lives will take place in cyber space – without the need for direct contact.

We will not have to leave our living room couch to do many of our daily chores. If what many experts are predicting turns out to be true, then the Internet and television will become one: a gigantic information box with which we will be able to receive and distribute all communication we require from and to the outside world.

4. The Mobile Trap

In 1998 over 160 million mobile phones were sold throughout the world. One in two Austrians, 20% of all Germans, 58.5% of all Finns and 54% of all Swedes use mobiles. These numbers are even higher in the U.K. and U.S.

The market is far from saturated. Sixty percent of all mobile phone users are men. The markets of the future, therefore, are women and children. According to a study undertaken by the Austrian Market Research Institute, 94% of those under 30 find mobiles "cool." We are on the way to becoming a mobile society; perhaps we are already there.

> *94% of those under 30 find mobiles "cool."*

No other electronic device reaches into our private lives as intensively as the mobile. The fear of missing out on something turns us into mobile telephone boxes, reachable 24 hours a day, always on stand-by. Mobiles are status symbols. They give us the feeling of being important, meaningful, and, above all, irreplaceable.

- Mobiles are addictive. Half of all messages sent via mobile are worthless.
- Mobiles create stress. We often telephone when our mind and heart actually need relaxation.
- Mobiles are becoming more and more powerful. It's not enough just to place a call. With a mobile you can now get access to the Internet and send e-mails and text messages.

I do not present you with these facts to scare you. Many of us have no problems with technological developments and most do not have to fear the future. But it is important to remember what I said at the beginning: technology must never be the master, it must always remain the servant.

Barnard Tips for a Healthy Heart
The 10 Best Rules to Avoid the Technology Trap

1 **Think positive.**
   Don't be afraid of new technology. Fear is always a bad counselor.
2 **Be critical.**
   Do you really need every new device, or do you just want to make an impression?
3 **Set limits.**
   You don't take your car into your bedroom, do you?
4 **Give your computer some time off.**
   Make an effort not to use your PC on certain days of the week.
5 **Forget your mobile.**
   Intentionally leave your mobile at home or in the office. This will help you to relax.

6 **Be the boss.**

You give the orders, not your mobile or your Internet connection.

7 **Don't force yourself to do anything.**

If you don't feel comfortable with technology, then don't use it.

8 **Stay single.**

Eat solo. Your mobile is not required as a dinner companion.

9 **More privacy please.**

Not everyone needs to know your e-mail address or your mobile number.

10 **Get up and move.**

Sport is not only fun to watch on television – participate.

13 Take Viagra

If you have a cold you take medication.
Why don't you do the same if you have
problems with sex?

A few months ago I was in Europe and perchance I glanced over a copy of the *Bild am Sonntag* newspaper. There I came across a story about me. After reading a few lines it was as if I had been struck by lightning. It said my wife had asked for a divorce because she had found condoms and Viagra in my travel bag.

The next day the telephone went wild. The whole world was apparently obsessed with finding out about my sex habits. How potent did I think a 76-year-old man should be? What was I like in bed? And last but not least, what was my true opinion of Viagra?

I have remained silent about these things because I am of the opinion that my private life should be respected and is nobody's business but my own. However, the wild rumors flying about from time to time have convinced me that it's time to clear a few things up.

It's true that Viagra was in my travel bag, but I have never taken it.

> *The Viagra in my bag was not for me but for a woman friend of mine.*

I don't know why my wife made such a big deal about it. We had separated some time previously. I had in the meantime moved from my home in Cape Town to another house. At the time she found the Viagra, we had already made the decision to go our separate ways. Perhaps my wife only wanted some degree of finality. I know that some people find it easier to detach themselves from a former loved one if they look for and exaggerate his or her mistakes. It helps them to distance themselves.

Actually I don't really understand all the commotion. First of all, it would have been easy to find out directly from me that I have never taken Viagra. On the other hand I have no qualms about people using any means they can to help with sexual problems.

I tell you this because I think we should rethink our approach to sex. If we have problems with our circulation then we consult a doctor. When we are ill we take medication. However, if we suffer from impotency we take nothing for it, and suffer in silence. We are ashamed to admit that we need help.

We live in a strange world. Everywhere around us there is sex, but no one really appears to want it that much. Sex is in ads, on TV, in magazines – but apparently nowhere in real life. Why is that? Is it because we are oversexed? Or because we suffer under extreme competitive pressures? Is it because we can no longer relax? Maybe it's because passion no longer fits into our "cool" lifestyle? Or could it be that we know everything about sex except how to enjoy it? Perhaps a little of all the above is true. However, the facts are:

- More and more men are impotent.
- Fewer and fewer women want sex.
- More and more couples are infertile.
- More and more people are looking for help through sex therapy.
- The sex aids business is booming.

I know of no other method which relieves stress as effectively as sex. You can sleep as much as you want, go to a health farm or indulge in relaxation exercises – nothing frees your mind or re-invigorates your soul like a satisfying love-making experience.

In Germany alone, 7.5 million men have potency problems.

This does not apply to everyone. For some people sex does not play a dominant role and they do not suffer because of it. In contrast, my whole life has been filled with passion – something I still have today. I have often experienced, both as a doctor and as a friend, how men take impotency to heart. The loss of virility is not comparable to any other kind of stress. Men are proud, they lose their dignity when they can no longer perform adequately.

Impotence is treacherous. It approaches very quietly, attacks suddenly, and refuses to let go. Once you cannot perform in bed, the next time creates such pressure that the next flop is virtually programmed.

> *A diabolical cycle: impotency puts you under extreme pressure and this stress manifests itself in your impotence.*

Impotency is no longer a malady affecting a small group. An estimated 140 million men around the world suffer from this affliction. The Massachusetts Male Aging Study found evidence that one in every two American males between the ages of 40 and 70 has erection problems on occasion. Ten percent of those studied were completely impotent.

Two-thirds of all men over the age of 60 no longer find sex satisfying. And even 7.5% of males between 20 and 40 suffer erectile dysfunction.

Impotency Begins in the Head

Impotency can have many causes – physical problems, illness, certain medications, drugs, smoking, and alcohol abuse to name just a few. In many cases, however, psychological problems play an important role. Sex is also always a state of mind. A mental block is the first step in the direction of impotency.

For many men it would be easier if they could talk about their suffering. But sex is still a taboo subject and therefore millions of men walk around with a heavy heart not knowing what they can do about their problem.

But they can be helped. The best-known means of combating impotency is Viagra. It is probably not the best method and, after the initial euphoria, sales are rapidly dropping around the world. Viagra can cause various side-effects and cannot be used in combination with most other medications. It should not be used on patients with heart disease because it causes a drop in blood pressure.

There have been alarming reports about Viagra as a cause of death in various cases, but these accounts have not been scientifically verified.

No medication has been the subject of such intense interest as Viagra, which was originally developed as a heart and blood pressure medicine. Upon its introduction on May 27, 1998, the pharmaceutical company Pfizer sold 350,000 packs within the first three weeks. The value of company stock rose to $150 billion – a rise of 163%. It was the first time in history that (legal) sex made people into millionaires!

> *The Viagra boom made people into millionaires and may have helped to save the rhino from extinction.*

As strange as it may sound, Viagra may also have, indirectly, helped to prevent the extinction of the rhino. Until this sex pill came on the market, a remedy derived from rhinoceros horns was looked upon as the greatest aphrodisiac – an assumption that is nonsense, by the way, as the horn of these creatures is nothing but hair. The life of the rhino has become much quieter since Viagra became available.

But now things have also become quiet for Viagra. After selling 35 million pills in the United States and three million in Germany, a reality check has taken place. Pfizer has lost ground on the stock market. The news that more effective sex medication with fewer side-effects will be available soon has caused investors to spurn the company.

It is true that with the new millennium a whole array of new and effective medications and methods will be on the market to help combat impotency.

- Viagra: the active substance (sildenafil) in the blue pill activates the erectile tissue receptors in the penis, but has no effect on the pleasure centre of the nervous system. Therefore it is necessary to be sexually aroused in order to obtain an erection. Success ratio 70%.

> *Apomorphine – the new sex wonder weapon from the U.S. – also helps women.*

- Apomorphine: a new medication that is currently being clinically tested in the United States. It affects the central nervous system and therefore can also achieve results in women. Projected success ratio also about 70%.
- Prostaglandin: an active substance which men can inject themselves with – a so-called "potency shot" – directly into the penis. Sounds more unpleasant than it actually is, but it should only be applied with a doctor's consent. Success ratio again 70%.

In addition, natural substances are becoming more and more successful in the battle against impotency. A whole batch of preparations based on plant substances are presently being employed to preserve male virility. Ginkgo biloba, for instance, is obtained from the leaves of the ginkgo tree. Since first studies revealed that this substance can help every second male with potency problems, sales in the U.S. have virtually exploded. Nearly 11 million Americans are already convinced of the powers of this extract. The sales of ginseng products are going equally well since an increasing number of studies have ascribed a potency-heightening effect to this legendary root.

> *Does the solution to our sex problems lie in the bark of some tree? At least 10 million Americans already believe this.*

Admittedly a charming idea: perhaps the raw material for the next potency star on the stock markets can be found in your garden.

Barnard Tips for a Healthy Heart
The 10 Best Paths to a Satisfying Sex Life

1 **Enjoy sex.**
   Only those with a positive inclination towards sex will enjoy it.
2 **Stay relaxed.**
   Sex can only relieve tension if you are relaxed.
3 **Forget about your potency problem.**
   One in two men has had at least one problematic episode with his potency.
4 **Tell someone about it.**
   Talk to your friends about more than your job and your holidays.
5 **Be honest.**
   Don't lie to yourself about your sexual problems.
6 **Be forthright.**
   Your partner has a right to know that you want to, but can't.
7 **Sport is sexy.**
   If you're in good shape, you reach your goals in bed as well.
8 **Help yourself.**
   Treat continued impotency as you would a cold virus: consult your doctor.
9 **Go to a doctor.**
   Doctors can listen, be discreet, and know about medication that can help.
10 **No sex stress please.**
   Don't let trends dictate how often you want to – or have to.

14 Learn to Love Brahms

It doesn't matter if it's hard rock,
pop or classical music. Whatever
music you prefer can relax you.

Music has always made an immense impression on me. It can make me sad, soothe me, or put me in good spirits. A few days ago I was in the car and heard "Crocodile Rock" by Elton John on the radio again for the first time in a long time. It is one of my favorite songs and Elton John is one of my favorite singers. The music immediately affected my mood: from one minute to the next I was happier.

The latest research results confirming the enormous effect music has on us, therefore, come as no surprise to me. More and more studies show that music can not only provide help in therapy – where it has been successfully used for some time – but it can be an aid in daily life as well, to help relieve stress.

Music is part of our lives since birth. The first contacts between parents and child occur through tones, sounds, and noises. Parents attempt to convey a sense of security to their baby through the soothing sounds they emit. The child listens fascinated or tries, through squealing and babbling, to answer. Mechthild and Hannes Papousek from the Pediatric Institute in Munich have discovered that parents mimic the melodic patterns of their offspring. Parents, for instance, try to get the attention of their baby by making cooing-like sounds.

> *Music is a balm for the soul: it quiets us, takes our fears away, and is good for the heart.*

The research concerning the effect music has on us has been going on for quite some time now. It has been known for a long time that music influences our moods. It can put us in good spirits, anger us, or relax us. Now more studies seem to point out that music can do even more. It can give us strength, harmony, and health.

- Music stimulates creativity. Classical music listened to through headphones increases concentration. Distractions are tuned out.
- Music takes away fears. A U.S. study among heart attack patients shows that individuals who listen to music along with their therapy have less fear of their illness. A second study shows that the therapeutic effect of music increases the more it is used.
- Music reduces weight. Music provokes a reflexive urge to move. Dancing for 15 minutes to disco or pop music can burn up 100 calories.

> *When you work with music, you solve problems more quickly and precisely.*

- Music is good for the heart. A German study was able to provide evidence that music can particularly help people suffering from hypertension. Music was played to a test group: a Strauss waltz, a modern classical piece, and meditation music. The effect was the strongest on those in the study group suffering from high blood pressure. The levels of the stress hormone cortisol were reduced by listening to all three kinds of music.
- Music reduces stress. The renowned American Medical Association recently quoted a study that showed music to be particularly relaxing in stress situations. Fifty surgeons were given mathematical problems to solve. The group of doctors who had background music were faster and more precise in

their problem-solving. Their blood pressure and pulse rate were lower. The doctors worked even better when they were able to choose their own music.

There is another new finding as well: how we experience music – as relaxing or irritating – does not depend on the rhythm or sound level but depends solely on our taste. Dr. Susanne Hanser, director of Music Therapy at Berkeley College in Boston, established that our blood pressure and breathing rhythm remain the same regardless of whether we're listening to techno-rock or soft love ballads. If we like the music we're hearing, our body reacts positively.

Music can also be a good lightning conductor for aggressive feelings.

A study by Heiner Gemberis, professor of Music Science at the Martin-Luther University in Halle/Wittenberg (Germany), confirms these results. However it's not taste alone that decides if music gives us wings or brings us crashing to the ground. It is our current mood as well. Gemberis played a relaxing tape of birds chirping and waves breaking to a test group. At the same time, a second group was given a complicated set of puzzles. Afterwards both groups were played musical pieces of various kinds. The group played the relaxing sounds found most of the songs soothing; the stressed puzzle group, on the other hand, reacted aggressively to most of the music.

This confirms the effect music has on us:

- It can influence our moods.
- It can relax us.
- It can be a lightning conductor for our aggressions.

Everyone can experience this him- or herself. I love Country and Western and Dixieland music. Among my favourites are "Take the Ribbon from Your Hair," Billy Joel's "River of Dreams," and Elton John's "Nikita." These songs inspire me and give me a zest for life.

I cannot imagine what it takes to write a symphony.

I can't really get anything out of "techno," "house," or "garage" but I revere classical music. My mother played the organ and I learned how to play piano. Sadly I can't play anymore because of my arthritis. I love Chopin, Beethoven, and Brahms. One of the most memorable experiences in my life was when, many years ago, I was a guest at the Salzburg Festival. I can't imagine being able to compose a symphony. Perhaps some composers think the same way about heart surgeons!

15 Sleep at the Office

Thirty minutes of sleep at midday is
worth as much as two hours of sleep at night.

At first glance, my very heartfelt suggestion about how best to relax at work might seem a bit crazy: sleep. If you're the boss of a company you will ask me why you should pay someone to sleep on the job. If you're an employee you most likely will shake your head and say, "No time and I'd get the sack." To the head of the company I would like to give the following answer: "If you let your employees sleep, the amount of work-related accidents and incidents in your company will drop dramatically." To the employee I would like to point out: "Allow yourself a nap. You will be reinvigorated and bubbling with creative energy."

Fatigue at work is more widespread than originally thought.

- According to a study by the Institute of Social Medicine at the University of Vienna, almost 70% of women and 54% of men suffer from chronic fatigue.
- A survey in Germany revealed that 50% of those questioned had at least one attack of fatigue a day.

Three-quarters of all women and half of all men have attacks of fatigue at work.

- A research study in Sweden found that 85% of controllers at an oil refinery occasionally fell asleep while working. Sleeping on the job is a punishable offense in the company.

Something that is frowned upon in Germany is a way of life in some countries. In Spain the *siesta* is an integral part of daily life. In many Mediterranean countries, shops close at midday so that everyone can have their nap. And it is in the countries that allow for phases of recreation during the workday that the number of heart and circulation illnesses is astoundingly low.

In China every worker has the right to take a midday nap. It has been reported that Winston Churchill took frequent naps in order to enable him to cope with his enormous work schedule. It is said that Salvador Dali sat down and made himself comfortable in his desk chair every day for a nap, with a spoon in his hand. When the spoon fell on the floor he awoke and was full of inspiration.

The Ideal Nap

It is scientifically proven that naps between 10 and 30 minutes long can dramatically increase one's performance. A study in the U.S. found that a 30-minute nap at midday has the same value as two hours of sleep at night. According to the latest research, a nap at work increases our reaction and concentration abilities. An improvement in mood, memory, and heart function was also found to take place.

Here and there American companies have begun to provide their employees with recreational rooms for resting. In Britain and Germany, companies are not following this good example. The German trade union federation suggested a few years ago that nap times should be introduced in offices. But this suggestion was greeted with sarcasm and ridicule, and quickly withdrawn.

In the meantime, it's perfectly clear why we are more and more fatigued. It's because stress at work is increasing and time for recuperating is continually decreasing. Accidents at work cause millions in damage every year. Frequently, fatigue and deteriorating reaction times are the culprits. Many motorway accidents are the result of drivers falling asleep at the wheel.

While companies are not (yet) sending their employees to "dormitories" to take naps, many have discovered that employees' health is part of a company's assets. International conglomerates such as IBM and Coca-Cola started a few years ago to convey the importance of relaxation seminars to their top managers. Now British companies have also acquired a taste for relaxation.

> *People not doing any sport lose more working days to illness.*

This thinking is based purely on sound economics. According to a study by the Science Institute of German Doctors, employees who do not do any exercise miss an average of 10.1 days a year because of illness. Sporty workers in the same age bracket miss only 8 days.

This should serve as a wake-up call. The German financial weekly *Wirtschaftswoche* recently found out that more and more companies are recommending exercise programs for their labor force.

- From 6.30 a.m., BMW offers its employees an "Early Wakeup." In two company-owned fitness centres, pre-work exercise programs are offered for employees.
- Daimler-Chrysler also provides its employees with two fitness and health centers located on the plant grounds.
- At Munich's Public Transport Services, bus drivers are sent regularly to psychologists and physical education instructors for training sessions. This procedure was instituted after findings obtained in 1993 showed that overworked drivers become unfit to drive.

> *At BMW the working day starts at 6.30 a.m. with an "Early Wakeup."*

- The German TV network RTL prescribes a special sports program as part of re-education sessions. The cost for each associate amounts to 2,000 marks.
- Companies such as Siemens, Lufthansa, and Porsche grant their top management "Wellness weekends" to relax.

According to the *Wirtschaftswoche*, most companies run up against an unexpected hurdle in their attempts to promote a healthier environment: their employees. Many are only prepared to accept the sports activities after intense consultations. They're afraid of harming their careers if they don't work continuously.

16 Take Some Quality Time Off

The best thing you can do for your health
and your career: take a three-week holiday.

A while ago I ran into a medical colleague of mine at an airport. He is a few years older than me and also quite well known since one of his patients is Boris Yeltsin. We spoke briefly and I asked him if he was still practicing medicine. "Yes," he answered. "What else can I do?"

At first this response confused me because I had had no trouble quitting my profession. One day I woke up and no longer had the desire to be a doctor. So I quit.

Later, as I sat on the plane, I mulled over my colleague's response and all of a sudden I realized why he'd answered as he did: many of us have forgotten how to let go.

We find it difficult to give up the jobs we have become accustomed to. We have difficulty giving up the work we have done most of our adult lives and go into retirement. And it has become increasingly difficult to leave our jobs during the year and take a real holiday we can enjoy. Just recently I read something very interesting: "It's no longer stress that makes us ill, but the lack of recreation."

The Hamburg Institute of Recreational Research has discovered that for more and more people a holiday is no longer relaxing but a burden. One in four develops an illness induced by "recreational stress." There are many reasons for this:

- We take the wrong holiday. More and more frequently we ignore the purpose of a holiday – to give us a balanced reprieve from work. If someone is under constant pressure during the year at work, it doesn't make sense to plan an action-packed holiday.
- We take too little time for our holiday. Only 7% take more than two weeks of holiday at a time. For 47% of people, the summer holiday lasts only 10 to 14 days. Forty percent of people only take a one-week holiday. A great many studies confirm that holidays should last at least three weeks in order to provide the right amount of relaxation.
- We race into a holiday. When offices and schools close, all the main highways are jammed. Yet most psychologists warn that such a sudden surge into a holiday is an unnecessary burden. At least two days should pass between the last day at work and leaving to go on holiday.
- We overvalue our holiday. Many feel it should be compensation for all they're missing throughout the year. Therefore holidays should provide rest, a bit of adventure, be educational, harmonize family life, and add more passion to one's sex life. These high expectations cannot be fulfilled by any holiday.

The most frequent mistake we make in our holidays: we try to make up for what we have missed during the year.

Apart from the computer industry, the tourist trade is the fastest growing industry in the world. Every year almost 500 million people are on the move as tourists. They spend, on average, approximately 13% of their disposable income. Over 100 million people around the world make a living, directly or indirectly, from the tourist industry.

The Brits are among the most globetrotting nations of all. And all-inclusive holidays are booming. Almost one in three takes a package holiday. The favourite destination is Spain. Millions flock to Mallorca and the Iberian beaches as if waved there by a magic wand.

Every Second Holidaymaker Is Stressed

However, what should give us strength for the rest of the year frequently ends in stress, anger, and disappointment. Half of all holidaymakers are unhappy with their holidays. Of those taking package tours, the ratio jumps to two-thirds. Forty percent complain about flight delays, 33% about bad hotel rooms, and 31% about noise.

During holidays, relationship problems escalate. The German news magazine *Focus* recently published a study which found that one in four couples have fights with their partner while on holiday. According to American psychologist Carin Rubinstein, 11% of American long-distance travellers return home depressed from "holiday blues."

There is no patent remedy for the right holiday. What amounts to perfect recreation for one person could be stressful for another. Most experts agree about one thing, though: a decisive factor in making your choice for a holiday is your daily routine during the year. The recreation researcher Henning Allmer at the Sports University of Cologne (Germany) has profiled four basic holiday types:

1 If you have a stress-filled job you should seek a peaceful, relaxing holiday, i.e., a holiday at an idyllic lake instead of a beach holiday at a busy resort.
2 If your job appears to be monotonous, you should try a sports-inclined holiday.

Action, swimming, hiking: there's an ideal holiday for everyone.

3 If you have to digest a certain amount of frustration you should try an adventure holiday.
4 If you're feeling drained you should try to relax by hiking.

When I was still practicing medicine I always tried to take a three-week holiday once a year. While I was working I was always on the move, therefore I was mostly very happy just to be able to relax at home. Just recently I read that this kind of holiday can provide better recreational value than a trip abroad. As part of a study in

Kiel, Germany, a group of teachers was sent to the beaches of southern Europe while another group stayed at home. The beach group quickly reflected the general relaxed feeling of contented holidaymakers in good spirits. However, after returning back to their jobs the absorbed energy was just as quickly spent and gone within three weeks. Those who stayed home took longer to get into a relaxed holiday groove, but then profited for the next 10 weeks and more from their three-week holiday.

The reason could be that many people have the wrong impression of what a holiday really means. It's more than just eating, drinking, and sunning yourself. A good, relaxing holiday deals with the whole body. Yet every second holidaymaker belongs to the lazy-holiday type. Lie on the beach, swim a bit, eat, and sleep. There's hardly time for more. But a recent study showed that switching off all intellectual activity during a holiday can temporarily lower one's IQ. So you should at least take the time to do a crossword puzzle.

Naturally, after months of hard work we feel the need to do nothing and chill out. But don't forget that the two big Bs need recreation as well: Body and Brain. The value of holidays without exercise or intellectual stimulation melts as quickly as ice in the southern sun.

Barnard Tips for a Healthy Heart
The 10 Best Tips for a Perfect holiday

1 The Glide Trick

   Glide slowly in and out of your holiday. Give yourself a two-day buffer between job and holiday. This helps avoid stress.

2 The Thursday Trick

   Return to work on a Thursday. Then your first week back is only two days long.

3 The Plane Trick

   Sit as near the front of the airplane as possible. There's less motion and the air is better.

4 The Hungry Trick

   .t's the best way to tell if your holiday was long enough. Ask yourself if you're eager to get back to work.

5 The Motivation Trick

Use the last days of your holiday to set yourself goals for the next few weeks. This gives you something to look forward to.

"Hungry" for your job again? Then your holiday was long enough.

6 The Breakdown Trick

Don't expect too much from your holiday. Reality is seldom as nice as the brochure makes it seem.

7 The Love Trick

Don't force your partner into a holiday. You might just then hear: "I didn't want to come here in the first place."

8 The Sport Trick

Those who exercise during a holiday return home in a better mood and also avoid having to diet.

9 The Sex Trick

Take your time. You can't catch up in one night what you missed the whole year.

10 The Planning Trick

Holiday crises occur most frequently on the third, seventh, and tenth day, of a holiday. Take this into consideration when planning your daily schedule.

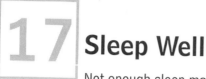

17 Sleep Well

Not enough sleep makes you weak,
sickly, and impotent. Too much raises
the risk of a heart attack.

My second wife, Barbara, always said, "For the Barnards, two things are important in life: love and sleep." Actually I have always spent a lot of time in bed, even when too much sleep was bad for my arthritis. I usually go to bed between 9 and 10 p.m. and get up at 7 a.m. to take my son to school. I once read that a 60-year-old man who sleeps eight hours a day has already slept away 20 years of his life. That scared me a little, because I've always been full of energy and have been intent on experiencing as much as possible.

Sleeping is the most sensitive form of relaxation. Our night's rest is the basis for our strength the next day. Every disturbance, be it noise or inner tension, has far-reaching consequences for the body. A person who over a long period of time cheats himself of sleep causes lasting damage to his body – even to the point of risking a heart attack.

> *You're 60? Then you have already slept away a third of your life.*

Because sleep has always been a basis of life it is relatively well researched. We know what happens to us while we sleep, which phases provide us with mental rest, and which provide the body with respite. As early as 1953 the pioneers of sleep research, Aserinsky and Kleitmann, were able to observe that at certain times during the night our eyes move up and down in jerky motions. They called these phases REM (Rapid Eye Movement) and differentiated them from non-REM phases, during which our eyes are presumably still. This opinion is still valid today.

Naturally, our knowledge of sleep has become more sophisticated over the years.

- We know today that our sleep begins with a non-REM phase, followed by sequences of REM and non-REM cycles, each of which lasts between 60 and 90 minutes.
- The REM phase serves as mental respite. During this phase we process most of the information and impressions we've gathered during the day. It is the time we have the most intense dreams.
- The non-REM phase provides the body with rest. This is when we sleep the deepest.
- The first non-REM phase contains most of our deep sleep. Therefore a disturbance here has the gravest consequences.

> *Don't fight nature: it has been genetically determined whether you are a morning or an evening person.*

Non-REM phases get shorter throughout the night. The REM phases, on the other hand, get longer. In layman's terms we say that as morning comes closer, sleep gets "lighter."

A good night's sleep is not a blessing sent by heaven. Our brain takes an active part in this process. A mechanism in our brain steers the change between non-REM and REM phases. In the meantime another mechanism in the brain directs our day and night rhythms.

Every person has different sleep requirements. It is genetically predetermined if we need a lot or very little sleep. Nature also determines if we are a morning or evening person. Everyone has to determine for him- or herself how much sleep is needed. A rule of thumb is that eight hours a night is generally enough.

Too much sleep is bad for the heart. For 10 years the Center for Disease and Prevention in the United States observed the sleep habits of 7,000 adults. The group that on average slept more than eight hours a day had a higher heart attack risk.

Less and Less Sleep

However, the much greater risk is too little sleep. The National Commission on Sleep Disorders Research in the U.S. estimates that 60 million Americans suffer from a chronic deficit. The average American sleeps approximately 20% less than his forebears a century ago. According to the experts, lack of sleep might be one of the biggest health risks we face today. As a matter of fact, many major accidents over the last years can be traced back to lack of sleep:

- The *Challenger* tragedy. On January 28, 1986, the space shuttle *Challenger* exploded shortly after takeoff. The ground crew was overworked; two of the most important members of the team had been awake for 19 hours straight before liftoff.
- The Chernobyl accident. On April 26, 1986, the atomic reactor in Chernobyl blew up. Millions were contaminated by the resulting radioactive fallout. An investigation showed that technical staff at the reactor had been chronically overworked.
- The *Exxon Valdez* catastrophe. On March 24, 1989, 11 million gallons of crude oil spilled into the ocean along the coast of Alaska. The ship's third mate, held responsible for the tragedy, had only slept for six hours in the two days prior to the accident.

Research at sleep laboratories has determined the following: a person sleeping an hour and a half less than he normally sleeps at night reduces his awareness by 33% the following day. A person who sleeps six instead of eight hours for two days reduces his reaction time by 10 to 15%.

> *A man who does not sleep enough reduces the oxygen flow to his penis.*

But the consequences for the body of sleeplessness go even further:

- **Less strength.** British weight-lifters who slept only three hours a night over three days suffered dramatic performance breakdowns on the second day.
- **Less growth.** During sleep the body produces 70% of the growth hormones it requires daily. A person not sleeping enough weakens his body's ability to strengthen muscle and bone.
- **Less immunity.** Men who sleep too little reduce the immune defence mechanisms of their body. This was determined in a research study at the University of San Diego.
- **Higher blood pressure.** A person who sleeps little has higher blood pressure during the day. A study in Japan determined this.
- **Less potency.** Automatic erection during the night ensures that blood is pumped into the penis. A man who does not sleep enough reduces the oxygen flow to his penis.
- **Less intellectual capacity.** People who suffer from sleep deprivation can have up to 25% less intellectual capacity.

Accidents which result from carelessness brought about by lack of sleep cause $46 billion in damages a year in the United States alone.

- **Less success.** Athletes who do not sleep enough lose more frequently. This was determined in a study at Stanford University.
- **Less fun.** A study at the Brigham and Women's Hospital in Boston showed that people who sleep according to their inner clock are happier and more balanced in their lives.

There are many things that can disturb our nightly rest – incorrect eating and drinking habits, noise or stress (more on this in Part III), psychological problems, etc. I usually sleep quite well, but if I have problems I sometimes lie awake for hours. This has happened a few times in my life. As I write this book, the divorce from my third wife is affecting me particularly deeply, and I have had great difficulty falling asleep over the past few months. Most of the time it has been impossible for me to get to sleep without taking a sleeping pill.

I think problems are the biggest reason for sleeping badly. All other factors, it would seem, at least have the possibility of a cure. Too much noise, too many cigarettes, bad eating habits can be dealt with. But sometimes we are powerless to deal with our problems.

> *If you fall asleep immediately upon lying down, you are not just tired but exhausted.*

Barnard Tips for a Healthy Heart
The 10 Best Ways to Sleep Well

1 Sleep is not a competition.
Taking 10 minutes to fall asleep is OK. If you regularly fall asleep the minute you hit the pillow, you're not tired – you're exhausted.

2 Pay attention to your inner clock.
It's better to sleep eight hours according to your body rhythm than 10 hours against your inner clock.

3 Don't count sheep.
If you haven't fallen asleep 30 minutes after lying down, get up and read a good book.

4 Smoke a peace pipe.
Altercations do not belong in the bedroom. Have a conciliatory talk with your partner before you go to sleep.

5 Don't sleep alone.
Separate beds are the first step to alienation. The exception to the rule: your partner snores.

6 Concentrate.
Why do we sleep? In order to relax and rest. Continue to tell yourself that.

7 Sleep according to a regular schedule.
Try to go to sleep at the same time every night. This programs your body to be prepared for relaxation.

8 Think positive.
A new day, new chances. Before falling asleep, look forward to the challenges of the next day.

9 Exercise.

Sport tires you out. But be careful: you should be finished with exercise four hours before you go to sleep.

10 No sleep orgies, please.

Don't try to compensate sleep deficits incurred during the week at weekends. Or do you breathe more on a Sunday too?

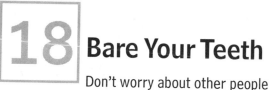

18 | Bare Your Teeth

Don't worry about other people
at work all the time. This causes
stress and harms your career.

Much in life is dependent on how we feel at work. Every day we spend about half our time in offices or some other workplace. If we experience this time as something positive, then the rest of our lives will be the better for it. If we experience our jobs as something agonizing, this creates stress, and this influences all other aspects of our lives.

It's a fact that an increasing number of people can no longer cope with the challenges posed at work. Conflicts in the workplace cause millions of dollars worth of damage every year. There are four major reasons for this:

1 Performance pressure. If you want success you feel you have to work harder and harder for it.
2 Technology. If you want to be on top of things, you feel you have to keep up-to-date with the latest innovations.
3 Career pressure. If it's a career you're after, everything else has to come second.
4 More competition. If you want to get ahead you must be able to hold your own at work.

Employees who don't feel comfortable at work are more frequently absent and work less than their contented counterparts. They are also sick more often. In the worst case scenario, they live with the fear of not being good enough and of possibly being considered for redundancy. This then causes them to feel uninvolved with their job, to do only as much as necessary, to sabotage any change in the regular work routine, and even to influence co-workers negatively.

Most managers don't even consider interfering with conflicts in the office. The result: an increasing number of us are suffering from job-related stress.

The vision of a friendly working atmosphere with fun co-workers who throw you a party on your birthday is looking more and more like an illusion. According to a new British study, the earlier you realize this the better you will adapt to your job. At work everyone is a lone warrior. The quicker one adapts to this fact, the better it is for one's career and for managing stress.

> *95% of employees believe that office politics have a greater influence on promotion than a good education.*

Psychologist Jane Clark discovered in the course of her research that hardly any employees believe there is any correlation between performance and career. Nearly 95% are of the opinion that office politics, cafeteria gossip, and hallway innuendo are the primary factors in career boosts. Education and efficiency, they feel, have little to do with it.

Clark has profiled three types of employee in her study:

1 Stars
2 Power People
3 Simpletons

Stars have the overview. They know what's going on around them. Their egos are always at the forefront and they are adept at creating alliances. However, their thinking is not exclusively egotistical. They often take on the role of leader. The success of an office or workplace frequently depends on how good Stars are at their job.

Power People think only of themselves and their careers. Everything else is secondary to their ambitions for success. They are prepared to lie and to manipulate others to achieve this. The workplace is just a vehicle they'll use to reach their personal goals.

Simpletons believe in the good in people. They seldom understand the power games going on around them. They believe in virtue, honesty, and sincerity. In the end, they are sure, justice will prevail. Simpletons most often lose out when it comes to promotion because they cannot make themselves the center of attention.

Office Intrigues – Join In

Jane Clark recommends keeping a cool head in the office. "Accept the fact that power games at the office are a part, albeit only one part, of your working environment. One has to learn to play this game well if one wants to get ahead. Many office workers want to keep out of office intrigues, but that seldom works. People with this attitude will always be left behind." In short: if it's a career you want, then you have to bare your teeth, throw your weight around, and be a clever tactician.

If someone is pressurized from all sides and doesn't learn how to deal with it, she not only loses out in the career chase, but also remains stuck on the first level. That person also endangers her health. This is the result of a study undertaken by the Volkswagen automobile corporation. The study contradicts the general opinion that it's top management who are prone to stress. For the study, workers were given blood pressure tests within a 24-hour time span. The results showed that 63% of the foremen suffered from hypertension.

Foremen are, not without reason, called 'vice-chiefs' (second-in-command) at VW. They have an immense amount of responsibility in production but very little space for individual decision-making: a frightening stress mix. The foremen are under pressure from two sides, above and below. A classic case of unmanageable stress.

Barnard Tips for a Healthy Heart

The 10 Best Weapons in the Power Struggle at Work

1 **Cool down.**

Don't try to smash down walls. You never know what's behind them.

2 **Praise yourself.**

Self-praise is nothing bad. After all, everyone should know how good you are.

3 **Learn to fly.**

Take a bird's-eye view of your office. This gives you perspective.

4 **Let off steam.**

Explode every now and then. A good thunderstorm can be very cleansing.

5 **Clench your fists.**

Confront office battles.

6 **Form a team.**

Surround yourself with capable people. This saves you a great deal of stress.

7 **Frustrated? Play a different game.**

Buy a video game. Your co-workers are not your personal punching bags.

8 **Establish goals.**

Knowing what you're fighting for makes it easier to cope.

9 **Share your stress.**

Find someone you can talk to about your feelings.

10 **Love in the office?**

Not a good idea. You don't take your desk home, so why take anything else home with you?

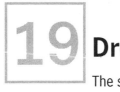

19 Drop Out

The simplest method to avoid stress
in your life: at least twice a day,
stop thinking about work!

How do you treat your car? Do you drive full speed until the engine explodes, or do you give it a break every now and then? Do you drive till the last drop of gas is gone or do you fill 'er up long before the tank's empty? Do you wait for the pistons to get stuck or do you check the oil? Don't treat your body any worse than your car. A person going full throttle around the clock is doing damage to body and soul.

Do you attack work as if you were driving 100 miles an hour all day? OK, but twice a day, pull over and get out. Because twice a day your body needs to regenerate:

1 when you're overworked and your mind can no longer cope with all the pressure
2 after work when you want to free your mind from the tensions of the day.

> *Don't treat your car better than you treat your body. Or do you always drive with your foot hard down on the gas pedal?*

There is no patent remedy for the right recreation after work. Everyone has to find out for him- or herself what the right method of relieving stress is for them. Some people enjoy sport, others like to meet up with friends, or just relax with the family. I always enjoyed gardening. The times I felt under pressure I found it soothing to see how my tomatoes were doing or what fruit tree was blooming. If I were more talented I would paint; fortunately I also had the ability to write. But as it is, gardening fulfils all my requirements for relaxation:

- It creates an inner peace, because stress and rushing have no place in nature.
- It takes place in the fresh air – balancing out all those hours spent behind closed doors at work.
- It frees the mind because it takes us away from the daily routine.
- It's inspiring: gardening is creative and nurturing.

Many people believe that they don't have time to relax. But relaxation is a vital part of the process. Perhaps you have experienced this for yourself: you sit concentrating for hours in front of your computer and then, after virtually forcing yourself to take a break, the best ideas come to mind.

What's the reason behind this? According to the medical psychologist Siegfied Lehrl from Erlangen (Germany), a person is particularly creative during times of rest. The mind is suddenly able to allow new visions to form and new combinations to evolve. Under pressure people are very goal-orientated but quickly lose their creative abilities.

> *The best ways to counter office stress: go for a walk or look out of the window for 10 minutes.*

It's so important that we pause to relax. I want to give you a few simple suggestions which can help you relieve stress in a matter of minutes while at work.

TIP 1 Get some air.

If your mind is blocked, get up and take a 30-minute walk. This will free your mind and break the mental block. The 30 minutes you "lose" by taking the walk you will quickly catch up with due to your reinvigorated mental capacity.

TIP 2 Do nothing.
Sit back in your chair and look out of the window (if you have one; if not, make a mental picture). Think of something completely different. Try to relax your entire body, concentrating on your breathing. This is a good way of relaxing.

TIP 3 Play golf in the office.
At first your colleagues might think you're a bit crazy. However, in the U.S. mini-golf sets for the office are all the rage. When nothing is working some managers now take a golf club in hand and putt around a little. This quickly clears one's thoughts because you are concentrating on something else. By the way, most of these office "putters" have never actually been on a real golf course.

TIP 4 Become a daydreamer.
Get comfortable, close your eyes and think of a place where you've been especially relaxed: on holiday, while engaging in sport or exercise, while on a walk or hike. This positive memory will lift your spirits.

TIP 5 Go for flower power.
Flowers can work wonders. Put a fresh bouquet of flowers on your desk, take a look at it every now and then, and enjoy its beauty. This will provide you with positive thoughts.

TIP 6 Read the writing on the wall.
Grab anything with lettering and hang it on the wall about 10 feet from your desk. Try to read something from it every half-hour; this relaxes the eyes.

TIP 7 Close your eyes.

Rub your hands together until they are warm. Put your hands gently on your eyelids and let your hands remain there for about three minutes. The warmth of your hands helps your eyes to relax.

TIP 8 Yawn a lot.

A little bit of magic. Yawning relaxes your facial muscles and automatically creates tear fluids in your eyes, keeping them from becoming too dry.

TIP 9 Bathe yourself in light.

Turn your face (eyes closed) towards the sun. Move your head slowly from side to side. This relaxes eyes and mind.

TIP 10 Stand up straight.

A simple trick. Make it a habit to get up every time you make or take a phone call. This relaxes the whole body and helps the circulation.

There are also some keep-fit exercises to combat stress in Part IV.

20 No Smoking, Please

Your last cigarette was yesterday.
If you really want to quit smoking,
then do it cold turkey.

I have never been a serious smoker. A few times when I had problems I smoked cigarettes: after a complicated operation or after the divorce from my second wife, Barbara. It's been 12 years since the last time I smoked. Today I don't even like it when people around me smoke, as it makes me have difficulty breathing.

Smoking is a strange habit. It's been known for decades what serious consequences it can have. It is one of the leading risk factors for heart and circulatory problems. Even though the Terry Report first warned about the dangers to health as a result of smoking some 35 years ago, the number of people smoking around the world is still astonishingly high. Although an increasing number of people in the Western world are giving up smoking, globally very little has changed. Smoking has been dramatically reduced in countries with intensive anti-smoking campaigns, like Great Britain and Norway. On the other hand, twice as many Africans smoke as compared to 1970.

Smoking is no longer a male thing. Already a quarter of all women are smokers. Among young people, more girls than boys are reaching for their cigarettes.

- According to estimates by the World Health Organization, one-third of the world's population over the age of 15 smokes; that's 1.2 billion people.
- Three-quarters of all smokers are in the developing countries. In China alone there are over 300 million smokers.
- Smoking is not only limited to men. In the industrial nations 42% of all men smoke, while the number of women smokers is steadily increasing, currently up to 24%.
- In Germany, 18 million people smoke. Every year 110,000 men and women die as a result of their nicotine habit. The German Anti-Smoking Initiative estimates the economic costs at 100 billion marks a year.
- Germany has the most young smokers in all of Europe. One in three girls smokes a cancer stick.
- Women are starting to take the initiative when it comes to smoking. Among 15-year-old boys, 21% smoke, but 29% of their female counterparts smoke. The "relapse quota" of women who have tried to quit smoking is over 50%, much higher than that of men, whose quota lies at 37%.
- In the U.S. and Great Britain, more women are dying as a result of smoking than from breast cancer.

Every 10 seconds someone, somewhere in the world is dying as a result of smoking. A report in the *European Respiratory Journal* stated that 500,000 Europeans die every year from smoking-related illnesses. That is many more than die from AIDS, suicide, hard drugs, car accidents, and guns combined. Cancer is still by far the leading cause of death from smoking. Lung cancer is four times as prevalent among women today than 30 years ago.

If it's clear how much damage cigarettes can do, why do people still smoke? Because it provides pleasure, gets our circulation in gear, or because it looks cool?

THE 10 MOST IMPORTANT ARGUMENTS FOR SMOKING

Argument 1: Smoking Is a Pleasure

Nicotine in a cigarette can be either stimulating or soothing. Smoking is frequently associated with terms such as "lifestyle," "recreation," and "relaxation."

Smoking is sexually satisfying. Our lips are erogenous zones which we stimulate with cigarettes.

Argument 2: Smoking Connects

Smoking can help make contact with others easier. Psychologically we show peaceful intentions when we offer someone a cigarette.

Argument 3: Smoking Relieves Stress

Smoking serves as a ritual for relaxation. The cigarette after work signals the beginning of leisure time.

Argument 4: Smoking Provides Security

Smokers have something to do with their hands when in company. Cigarettes give security and downplay insecurity.

Argument 5: Smoking Is Oral Satisfaction

The mouth and lips are erogenous zones. Smoking fulfils the same function as kissing.

Argument 6: Everybody Smokes

Parents, grandparents, siblings, and friends smoke, so we might as well light up too.

Argument 7: Smoking Is Cool

Ads depict smokers as happy, free, and adventurous individuals. That influences us.

Argument 8: Smoking Keeps You Thin

People who stop smoking gain weight. Eating is often a compensation for the lost pleasure of a cigarette.

Argument 9: Smoking Makes You Happy

Smoking influences your mood. Nicotine provides the smoker with a positive rush.

Argument 10: Smoking Increases Performance

The nicotine in a cigarette can stimulate us. It releases chemical substances called neurotransmitters within the brain.

... AND THE 20 MOST IMPORTANT ARGUMENTS AGAINST SMOKING

Argument 1: Smoking Makes You Sick

Cigarette smoke contains 4,000 different substances, many of which are harmful to the body. These include carbon monoxide, tar, cadmium, arsenic, and hydrocyanic acid. Smoking is a cause of cancer and a major risk factor for heart and circulatory disease.

Argument 2: Smoking Is Addictive

When nicotine levels drop, smokers light up. This cycle is what creates and sustains the dependency on cigarettes.

Argument 3: Smoking Damages the Heart

Cadmium and nicotine cause high blood pressure. Carbon monoxide decreases the oxygen content of your blood.

More than a third of all heart deaths are the direct result of tobacco consumption.

According to the W.H.O., 35% of all deaths from heart and circulatory diseases can be attributed to smoking.

Argument 4: Smoking Decreases Life Expectancy

The death rate in the age group between 35 and 54 is three times higher for smokers compared to non-smokers. Deaths attributed to tobacco occur 20 years earlier than the average.

Argument 5: Smoking Raises the Cholesterol Level

The carbon monoxide in tobacco smoke attacks the metabolism. It promotes the development of bad cholesterol (LDL) and inhibits the good cholesterol (HDL).

Argument 6: Smoking Reduces Performance

Constant intake of nicotine inhibits the nervous system and interferes with blood circulation and the flow of oxygen to the brain. This leads to a noticeable decline in performance.

Argument 7: Smoking Weakens the Immune System

Smokers have colds more frequently, and these can lead to major illnesses. The limited circulation and oxygen flow in the body inhibit the immune system.

Argument 8: Smoking Leads to Poisoning Symptoms

Smoking can cause headaches, sleeping disorders, paranoia, and digestive problems.

Argument 9: Smoking Disturbs the Sense of Taste

Tobacco smoke dries out the mucous membranes and damages the smell and taste receptors in the mouth and nose.

Argument 10: Smoking Causes More Harm to Women

Women who smoke and take the contraceptive pill have, according to a U.S. study, a 34-times higher than average heart attack risk.

Argument 11: Smoking Causes Impotency

A smoker reduces the blood circulation in his whole body. It's also speculated that the substances contained in cigarettes can reduce potency.

Argument 12: Smoking Reduces Birth Weight

Babies delivered by smokers are on average 9% lighter and 2% shorter; the head size is 1.5% smaller.

Argument 13: Smoke Gets in Your Eyes

In a research study done at the University of Tubingen (Germany), smokers were found to have more difficulty seeing blue and yellow on television screens. The reason? There is less blood circulation in the retina.

Argument 14: Smoking Makes Babies Aggressive

An Australian study speculates that children of smokers are more prone to aggressive behavior.

Argument 15: Smoking Hurts Everyone

According to reports from the W.H.O., passive smokers have a higher risk of getting heart disease and cancer.

Argument 16: Smoking Is Expensive

A person who forgoes his daily packet of cigarettes saves approximately $25,000 over a 10-year span – enough to buy a car or take several really good (three-week!) holidays.

Argument 17: Smoking Is a Role Model

Anyone who smokes is a bad role model for children. Children of smokers have an above average tendency to smoke themselves.

Argument 18: Smoking Causes Fatigue

The cadmium in tobacco smoke causes chronic fatigue. Random doses of nicotine can stimulate; a constant amount inhibits the system.

Argument 19: Smoking Ages

Smoking disturbs the circulation of the skin. That makes people look older earlier.

Argument 20: Smoking Is Out

Perhaps the most effective argument: in the Western world, at least, smoking is becoming less and less trendy.

It's a fact that smoking can severely damage the heart. Smoking more than 20 cigarettes a day brings with it a six-times higher heart attack risk. Combine this with another risk factor such as high blood pressure and the chances of an illness do not double, they quadruple.

Over the course of the past years the number of treatments for smoke addiction has increased dramatically. Today, if someone really wants to quit smoking they can. There is a multitude of therapies and remedy products such as nicotine patches and nicotine sprays. Also available are an array of psychological support groups.

> *There have never been so many types of treatment for addiction to smoking available as there are today. Anyone who really wants to can rid themselves of this vice.*

I am still of the opinion that the most successful method of quitting smoking for most people is cold turkey (stop abruptly and don't start again). My third wife, Karin, stopped smoking in one day. She had a cold and all of a sudden smoking no longer gave her pleasure. So she stopped and has not smoked a cigarette since.

There are five effective methods of quitting:

1. The Abrupt Method (cold turkey). You quit once and for all.
2. The Alternative Method. You support your efforts with acupuncture, acupressure and/or homeopathy.
3. The Psychological Method. You wean yourself from the habit with psychological support. Anything from hypnosis to autosuggestion.
4. The Substitute Method. You don't smoke cigarettes but give the body nicotine in short phases via chewing gum or patches.
5. The Pharmaceutical Method. You break the habit with the help of medication.

The New Superdrug

In the U.S. a drug called Zyban is currently being successfully employed. It blocks certain "messenger" substances in the brain, thereby reducing the longing for a cigarette. Studies have shown that Zyban can help many smokers who have previously attempted to stop smoking. In a comparative study, 38% successfully stopped smoking, more than double the number in the group using an ineffective placebo. But Zyban does have side-effects: feelings of nausea, headache, and dryness of the mouth.

Zyban is more successful when used in combination with nicotine substitutes. This relatively new form of therapy attempts to slay the enemy with its own weapons. Over a short span of time, smokers are not weaned from nicotine but actually receive it. Compensation for sacrificing the pleasures of cigarettes takes the form of a small dose of nicotine administered to the habit-breaker through the nose, skin or mouth. This provides the body with a certain level of nicotine and reduces the withdrawal symptoms.

SMOKER CHECK: HOW ADDICTED ARE YOU?

Taking the so-called Fagerström Test is the quickest way of determining the extent of your nicotine addiction. This test is most often used before the start of nicotine replacement therapy. Just add up the points to see how you score.

The five-minute Fagerström Test: find out how dependent you are on your cigarettes.

Fagerström Test

When do you smoke your first cigarette after getting up?

Within 5 minutes	3
6–30 minutes	2
31–60 minutes	1
after 60 minutes	0

Do you find it difficult not to smoke in places where it is specifically not allowed (i.e. church, libraries, the movies, etc.)?

Yes	1
No	0

Which cigarette would you be least willing to forego?

| The first one in the morning | 1 |
| Other | 0 |

How many cigarettes do you smoke a day?

Up to ten	0
11 to 20	1
21 to 30	2
31 and more	3

Do you smoke more in the morning than the rest of the day?

| Yes | 1 |
| No | 0 |

Do you smoke when you're ill and have to stay in bed?

| Yes | 1 |
| No | 0 |

Now add up your points.

0 to 2 points	A very low nicotine dependency
3 to 4 points	Low nicotine dependency
5 to 10 points	Medium to high nicotine dependency

There are various possibilities for nicotine substitution therapy: nicotine gum, nicotine patches, nose spray, inhalers, or nicotine pills. Which method is the best for each individual depends on what type of smoker you are and your degree of dependency on cigarettes. "Dosage smokers" feel the need always to keep the same level of nicotine in their system. Therefore they smoke relatively regularly throughout the whole day. A nicotine patch or an inhaler can best help them, since both products keep nicotine levels constant. So-called "High" smokers tend to smoke only at certain times (when under stress). They should try nicotine gum or a nose spray since they require a quick rush of nicotine to be satisfied.

> *Coordinate your stop smoking regime with a program of sporting activities. That will increase your chances of success.*

Whatever forms of therapy you choose, remember one thing: a therapy can only be successful if you change your lifestyle. Just cutting out cigarettes won't work. If you stop smoking and at the same time start an exercise programme, your chances of success increase rapidly. New studies confirm that a combination of withdrawal therapy and exercise makes it easier to quit smoking.

Barnard Tips for a Healthy Heart
The 10 Best Methods to Stop Smoking

1 **Stop immediately.**
   A 30-year-old man who quits has the same life expectancy as a non-smoker.

2 **If you have to, then make it light.**
   Fifteen milligrams less tar in the cigarette cuts the risk of a heart attack in half.

3 **Ladies first.**
   Women who smoke have a much higher heart attack risk than men.

4 **Exercise.**
   A U.S. study confirms that smokers who exercise can lower their heart attack risk.

5 **Smoke a pipe.**
   Converting from cigarettes to a pipe lowers the risk of a heart attack.

6 **Don't smoke a pipe.**
   ... but it's still 50% higher than non-smokers.

7 **Live longer.**
   A 30-year-old who has smoked for 15 years has a 6-year lower life expectancy – unless he stops smoking immediately.

8 **Don't overestimate yourself.**
   There are people who stay healthy despite smoking, but sadly we don't know which ones.

9 **Don't worry about weight gain.**
According to several studies, a weight gain of 5% is normal while quitting, anything more is purely a result of trying to feed your oral habit.

10 **Quit on-line.**
Even the Internet can help you to stop smoking. Every Thursday therapies begin on-line. The program takes a week. You can sign on anytime. The address: www.mdx.ac.uk/www/iqfl

Environment

21 Avoid Noise

Recent studies have shown that noise
has now become the second most
serious risk factor for the heart.

I cannot understand how an event like a Formula One race can attract millions of people – live and on television. According to the latest studies, every healthy person should actually instinctively get the urge to flee from such events. In the arena of those ever-so-sensitive four-wheeled rockets, every form of noise-measuring device will be destroyed. Anyone who has ever stood next to such a monstrous marvel of motoring while the drivers rev up their engines will know what I'm talking about. The screeching, almost malignant whine of the engines doesn't only cause pain to the ears but literally attacks the stomach, head, and heart – something which you can measurably feel in other parts of the body. I just can't understand why so many people put themselves in so much danger. One thing has for quite some time been established by scientific research even though the public has apparently not realized it yet: after cigarettes, noise is the second major cause of illness.

Only smoking puts your heart at more risk than noise does!

According to Hartmut Ising, the German physicist and press representative of the German State Institution for Earth, Water and Air Hygiene in Berlin, "Noise is the second biggest cause of heart attacks, a problem that up until now has been largely ignored or underestimated."

German researchers began gathering evidence on the effects of noise almost 20 years ago. They established two basic types of body reactions to noise: a passive form, which reacts with frustration to the influence of our surroundings, and an active form, which leads to confrontation or flight from the situation. In both cases the body increases production of stress hormones. In the passive form the stress hormone in question is cortisol; in the second form it's adrenaline and noradrenaline. In both cases the overproduction of these substances has negative effects on our health.

> *The body reacts to unexpected, unpleasant loud noise with fright and the increased production of cortisol.*

It is interesting to note the tests Ising employed with a study group in order to establish the effects of noise. He examined three levels of noise with the test group to see their varying reactions.

In this test he confronted one group of people with the engine noise of a Formula One race. The second group was confronted with loud noise kept at a continual level. The third was subjected to noise made by low-flying jets.

The results of the test showed that the noise of a Formula One race releases adrenaline into the circulation, because the so-called "central command" of the ear, just to be on the safe side, interprets the loud and unusual noise as a "danger." With noise that is continual, the body releases an excessive amount of the stress hormone noradrenaline. And the body reacts to a loud and unpleasant sound (the low-flying jet noise) with a sense of alarm and the feeling of impending danger, thus releasing cortisol.

The Dangerous Hormones

Summarizing the three tests, one can only come to the conclusion pointed out a few times in other parts of this book: noise increases the risk of a heart attack. Adrenaline and noradrenaline have negative effects on the immune system, the metabolism, cardiovascular system and blood composition (it gets "thicker"). An excess of cortisol will raise blood pressure. These changes occur even if the person appears outwardly to have adapted to the "noise pattern."

People, of course, possess different degrees of sensitivity, therefore their reaction to their surroundings can vary. I will now describe only three types of noise that can cause illness. These are ordinary noises with which we can be confronted at any time. They are:

1 Traffic noise
2 Noise from natural catastrophes
3 Noise which we generate.

Traffic noise from routine daily traffic, which today is hardly noticed by those subjected to it (people have got so used to it), endangers the health of millions of people in the Western world. This noise – hardly noticeable to many people any more – has its part to play in a phenomenon of our civilized times: people are fleeing whenever they have the chance into nature, but above all to a quiet, idyllic setting.

> *Anyone awakened by an earthquake risks a heart attack.*

Recently I came across a research study about the noise caused by natural catastrophes, noise which has varying effects on humans. The American physician David L. Brown of the Albert Einstein College in New York conducted the study. He investigated a combination of adult stress and strong emotional stress, termed "super-effect." He examined the data on two earthquakes in the U.S.: The Loma Preta quake that occurred on October 17, 1989 at 5.04 p.m., shaking San Francisco, and the Northridge quake, which occurred at 4.31 a.m. on January 17, 1994 and shook Los Angeles residents out of their sleep.

110 PERCENT MORE HEART ATTACKS

The statistics for heart attacks remained close to average during the first quake, however it rose to an unbelievable 110% during the second quake. This is astonishing when one remembers that the San Francisco earthquake was much more severe. I would assume that the population was under the same stress conditions in both California cities. The only difference quite obviously is the different times that the earthquakes occurred. While the people of San Francisco experienced the earthquake during office hours, the LA residents were literally shaken out of their sleep – the result was an increase of 110% in heart attacks. Robert Kloner, a cardiologist at the University of Southern California and a victim of the LA quake, later stated: "It was a big bang and sounded like an underground bomb explosion." It could therefore also be that the noise was an important contributing factor in the alarming increase in heart attacks.

My theory is supported by a study done by Arthur Wilde of the University of Amsterdam. He examined 11 families suffering from certain gene defects which resulted in an irregular heartbeat and life-threatening heart rhythm disturbances – called QT syndrome. The reason for the study was five unusual deaths, among them that of a 22-year-old man who apparently was so startled by his alarm clock that he went into cardiac arrest.

> *My favorite noise is the thunder before a storm.*

The results of Arthur Wilde's research – taking into consideration hereditary influences – can be formulated in one sentence. He proved without a doubt that for these patients every form of noise – from alarm clocks to bells and ambulance sirens – could be life-threatening, leading to cardiac arrest at any time. The best evidence: just 10 seconds after one member of the test group was awakened by an alarm clock at 3 a.m., serious heart rhythm problems set in. This could have proved fatal without the presence of a physician.

Not all noises are unpleasant. I myself am particularly soothed by three types of sounds:

1 thunder
2 the laughter of a child
3 the soft sounds of pleasure which a woman makes during sex.

I will explain why I mentioned thunder first. I grew up amid the endless expanse of South Africa's inland plains. That is why even today I still own a farm situated about 350 miles from Cape Town. We were frequently plagued by drought in that part of the Karoo and it often used to happen that sheep died of thirst and you used to find dozens of them lying shrivelled up on the dusty plains. When the rains finally came, they were always preceded by thunder. That thunder used to bring me a feeling of immense relief. Hence my love for this heavenly sound.

But I must admit that there is a sound that I can't stand. Whenever it occurs I withdraw as fast as I can: someone discussing his business for everybody to hear in a hotel foyer or airport lounge. It makes me long to be in a place where I can hear "the sound of silence."

Above all it is important to be able to shield oneself 100% from noise during one's time of rest. There is nothing that influences the value of sleep as much as noise. Even if one is not awakened by the noise, it can still do severe damage to one's health. As we know, the cardiovascular system is severely impaired by lack of sleep, and blood pressure rises to dangerous levels under these circumstances. One more thing: although the ear has a pain tolerance level of about 120 decibels, people frequently cannot tolerate a constant "noise pitch" – which is barely heard – for any length of time, even though it may be as low as 80 decibels. This too is a health risk.

> *"One day we will have to combat noise just as relentlessly as the plague."*

The great turn-of-the-century physician, Robert Koch was not only a brilliant bacteriologist but also a man of prophetic abilities. The 1905 Nobel prize winner already suspected in his time that: "One day people will combat noise just as relentlessly as cholera and the plague." This physician, who discovered the causative agents for tuberculosis and cholera, would perhaps even today be looked at somewhat disparagingly by a large number of people because of this statement.

Yet researchers in the area of noise pollution have been aware of the problem for some time. The aforementioned Hartmut Ising, of the German State Institution for Earth, Water and Air Hygiene, has accumulated hard facts for Germany and Europe:

- Exposure to constant noise affects people's lifestyle. They live with the windows closed, are less able to concentrate, and suffer from headaches more frequently.
- Eighty million people in Europe are severely threatened by traffic noise.
- In Germany alone over 60 million people are angered by traffic noise that disturbs their sleep, mostly at night.
- Noise is a contributing factor in 2,000 deaths annually in Germany.
- Traffic noise can raise the heart attack risk by 10%.
- Little or no noise at work would reduce the heart attack risk by 16%.
- Millions are exposed to noise levels at work that can damage their health.
- Hearing loss caused by excess exposure to hazardous noise levels constitutes 30% of work-related illness. These hearing-impaired workers receive occupational disability benefits amounting to millions a year.
- Improved noise protection could spare hundreds of thousands of people a year from the dangers of life-threatening cardiovascular problems.
- The Berlin audiologist Harmut Berndt maintains that if this trend continues, "a third of all youth will need a hearing aid by the time they are 50."

When you smoke you can stop, but can you do anything about the noise you are plagued with? To a large extent you can't – because a large portion of the public has not developed any sensitivity toward noise. Noise doesn't bother them or they try to ignore it, grossly underestimating its potential to cause damage. Rainer Guski, a professor of psychology at the University of Bochum in Germany, is of the opinion that the most important aspect of noise prevention and protection is "to make the public aware of the benefits." If noise reduction is not perceptible, then it will not be of any use.

> *We can do nothing about noise 90% of the time.*

Coupled to this is the fact that we are, in any case, unable to do anything about most of the noise that we are exposed to. People living near traffic arteries must either accept the noise or go and live somewhere else.

Private noise-prevention technology is usually very expensive. The Federal Environmental Agency in Berlin has estimated that fitting a sound-proof door, for example (which would result in a noise reduction of 4 decibels in a house or apartment) can cost twice as much as fitting a normal door.

Be that as it may, research has shown precisely when noise really leads to measurable damage to hearing: 85 decibels of noise at work leads, after 10 years, to at least a 30-decibel hearing loss. How the heart is affected can only be speculated about, but not measured. But you can assume that a constant noise level of even just 40 decibels will damage your heart. This is based on the assumption that you are annoyed by the noise or have other negative feelings about it.

Noise Is Experienced by the Individual

I think Professor Guski is right when he says that noise reduction has to be perceived in order for it to bring about a positive effect. Because noise can – in particular in the lower decibel levels – only be measured physically. When do we experience a noise as a nuisance? When is it still pleasurable – even though it may be loud. Just think about the various ways people experience sounds, like the difference between a dripping tap at night and the chirping of a bird in nature. Professor Guski is of the opinion that people do not feel comfortable in complete silence either, that they need "sounds to orient [themselves] in [their] surroundings."

> *What is noise? For some it can be a dripping tap!*

I am of the opinion that moments of absolute quiet can certainly do their part to assist in the cleansing or inner healing of a person. Therefore, my recommendation: try as often as you possibly can to escape the noise pollution of your surroundings. Take a walk in nature and surround yourself with its sounds (birds singing, crickets chirping, etc.) and you will reduce your heart attack risk.

22 | Don't Smoke, Even Passively

You think that smoking is dangerous?
It is. But so is passive smoking.

There are reasons why Americans so rigorously – often seemingly to the point of absurdity – take action against smoking in public places. Today it has been scientifically confirmed that active smoking is the highest health risk factor, but, as further research has shown, passive smoking has detrimental effects on health as well. This is the reason for the draconian punishments for people who ignore bans on smoking in public. It seems likely that soon smoking will not be allowed in public at all. Hallelujah.

The smoker is a species which is fortunately in danger of becoming extinct. In California a general smoking ban was initiated in bars and, recently, the first studies examining the results were released. In San Francisco 53 waiters were examined by Dr. Mark Eisner before and after the new regulations. The findings showed that 78% of the employees reported an improved physical sense of well-being four months after the implementation of the ban. Irritations such as burning in the eyes and breathing problems were simply "blown away." Mark Eisner and his team are sure that further anti-smoking laws and regulations can help reduce risks, particularly among those who are forced to inhale passive smoke.

How tennis superstar Andre Agassi stopped my wife from smoking.

It's not so long ago that I sat in an elegant Cape Town restaurant with my third wife, Karin, and a small group of friends. At the next table sat a world-famous couple: the tennis player Andre Agassi and his wife at the time, Brooke Shields. The couple's presence did not go unnoticed. At our table we were in the best of spirits, so much so that Karin, who was not a regular smoker, and some of our friends lit up.

Within a short time a waiter approached our table and – somewhat abashedly – asked us whether we would mind putting out our cigarettes. The request had come from the couple at the next table, Agassi and Shields. "Americans," he muttered and shrugged apologetically.

In many U.S. studies it has been established and widely publicized in the media that passive smoking can lead to cardiovascular problems faster than active smoking. During regular, active tobacco consumption defensive mechanisms can be developed over the course of time that cause a different "response" in the vessels, while non-smokers are unprepared and therefore virtually poisoned.

The Death Statistic

According to university professor Stanton Glanz, the author of over 80 studies concerning this subject, "Smokers continually challenge their cardiovascular system to defend itself against the regular supply of poison." Non-smokers do not do this, of course. This is the reason why indirect (passive) cigarette smokers have a lower ability to carry oxygen in their blood. The heart is subjected to stress, and the risk of a heart attack is even greater, because smoke activates cells that can cause blood to clot. According to Glanz's figures, approximately 47,000 Americans die annually as a result of passive smoke.

The American tobacco industry – having to deal with enough problems already – considers Glanz public enemy no.1 and calls him "the most militant non-smoker in the United States whose research is in stark contrast to other well-founded scientific studies."

47,000 Americans die annually from inhaling someone else's smoke.

138

I, however, feel that the desperate tobacco corporations will have no choice but to accept the fact that passive smoking is a risk factor for heart disease, because this conclusion has also been reached in studies done by highly acknowledged European research institutes. In a combined study by the Royal Medical School of London, the St. Bartholomew School, and the Wolfson Institute of Preventive Medicine, a team under the direction of Professor Wald came to alarming conclusions concerning passive smoking. The results of 19 separate studies conclusively showed that people forced to work or live with a smoker had a 30% higher risk of developing heart disease.

Even when the passive smoker is subjected to only one cigarette per day he runs the same risk as a person smoking nine to ten cigarettes a day. By the way, a person smoking only one cigarette a day increases his health risk by 39%.

The most damaging argument was revealed by the findings of Jiang He, a statistician at Tulane University. He was able to obtain 650,000 pieces of data from 18 relevant research studies from around the world (participating countries: Italy, New Zealand, China, England, Japan, U.S., Scotland) which he then analyzed by computer. The results showed that the health risk for cardiovascular diseases rises by 23% when a non-smoker lives and works in the vicinity of a smoker.

These results were greeted with a great deal of satisfaction at the University of Louisiana. This university is considered the cradle of all research concerning the consequences for health as a result of passive smoking. And Professor Gray Malcolm, a pathologist, regards the aforementioned percentage reached by his colleague Jiang He as too low. He speculates, without the benefit of evidence from a scientific research study, that the risk to passive smokers is even higher than currently believed.

> *I also smoked. It all began with dried donkey manure.*

All My Wives Smoked

I must admit that I have been aware of the risks of smoking for a long time, but I can't oppose it as vehemently as others. The reason for this is simple. I once smoked myself. It all began at the tender age of eight or nine. In those days, and at that age, smoking a cigarette seemed a terribly manly and grown-up thing to do. Not having the necessary finances, we were forced to go for a home-made version. We collected dried-out donkey manure, rolled it into pieces of old newspaper, and lit it. These were our first cigarettes.

My three ex-wives were all smokers. One smoked more, the other, Karin, smoked less. The cigarette I liked best was always the one after I had performed an operation. That cigarette seemed to relax me. I'm not sure what makes smoking so attractive. Perhaps it's just a subliminal memory of the time when we were babies and totally focused on our mother's breast.

Be that as it may, I gave up smoking twice. After my second divorce early in the 1970s, I began smoking again. A lot. Of course I was aware of the fact that smoking is dangerous. Nevertheless I only stopped smoking years later. I had an Australian girlfriend in those days. One day she implored me to stop smoking and I put out that cigarette and never lit another. Today, 20 years later, I must admit that smoking irritates me tremendously.

Smoking is probably the greatest risk factor for a heart attack. Passive smoking is surely very unpleasant, because you yourself can do little to prevent it. If you have a smoker as a partner, you can only hope to make them consider or understand your side of the situation. If you have a smoker as a work colleague, there is also very little you can do. But perhaps you can appeal to your boss to designate smoke-free zones at your premises. This would also be to the benefit of your company, as a reduced amount of sick leave could very well result from such a step.

> *Every non-smoker who works alongside a smoker is risking his or her own health.*

Barnard Tips for a Healthy Heart
Ten Ways to Deal with Passive Smoking

1 Go away.
   Simple but effective. Simply refuse to work with a smoker in the same office.

2 Offer some chocolate.

Perhaps you will succeed in getting the smoker to put your chocolates into his or her mouth instead of cigarettes.

3 Begin to smoke yourself.

Smoke for a few days and then stop. This may set an example.

4 Smoke cigars.

Strangely, cigarette smokers don't much like cigar smoke.

5 Read magazines for men/women.

Perhaps the smoker is prepared to exchange his/her cigarettes for your magazine.

6 Be ambitious.

Try to make a quick career of it and then, when you're at the top, ban smoking in your firm.

7 Play therapist.

Try going on the psycho-tour, talking through with the smoker why he/she smokes, and offering to help him or her quit. If it seems to work, you can ask to be paid next time.

8 Try fainting.

Study a few old Hollywood favourites – soon enough you too will be able to pass out in style.

9 The horror of it.

Learn the 10 most horrible consequences of smoking by heart and bombard the culprit with them vigorously.

10 Forget your manners.

Cutting your finger- or toenails, or picking your nose in the office, will send the smoker running away from you.

23 Consider Your Workplace

Money and prestige are important
in your job. But you should think
about re-arranging your office.

D o you remember when you bought your first home? You spent weeks looking at ads in the papers. You may have made hundreds of telephone calls, finding out about costs, locations, and prices. You wasted hours looking at prospective homes which didn't turn out to be what you were looking for at all. And further hours were spent in the offices of lawyers and real estate agents in the hope of making a flawless purchase.

But when you accepted your present job, how important was it for you to find out the conditions under which you were to be housed? Your job interview probably contained no mention of your workplace. But then your new boss took you to see your new office and you quickly sized it up, roughly estimating its size and what that implied about your position in the company.

> *You spend weeks looking for a new home. But what about your work surroundings?*

While we're dealing with accommodation here: you have slipped up badly. Just think for a moment of how much time you spend in your office and how much at home. You develop exact criteria for your home – and none for your place of work? You should not let that happen again.

142

Take smoking, for example. Perhaps you put up with it for the first few weeks. Live and let live. Let him smoke; he's a pleasant guy otherwise. But then, after a month perhaps, you get upset about it for the first time. You don't ask him to stop smoking altogether at first. "That's not what I mean," you hasten to add, untruthfully. "I'm only asking you to cut down a bit." He may make an effort but he will definitely be affronted, whether he says any thing or not. A few weeks later you have a complicated piece of work to finish and he's sitting opposite you, puffing away like a chimney. You give him a piece of your mind – and that's the end of your good working relationship.

Don't let them put you into an office with a smoker in the first place. You can't do that? Usually you can, you just have to be firm enough. Go to your boss and suggest the possibility of another seating arrangement or another room allocation. This is a good test. If your boss respects you, she will listen. If she really respects you, you will soon be sitting in a smoke-free workplace. If she doesn't care, look elsewhere.

> *A total ban on smoking in the workplace: 10 billion cigarettes would stay in their packets.*

Several research studies in Britain have found conclusive evidence that the risk of heart attack increases by 25% for a non-smoker in a smoking environment. Another British study found that 2% of all heart attacks are triggered by the constant inhalation of environmental poisons such as dioxin and black smoke in Britain's most polluted cities. The scientists concluded that if the environment were more healthy, 6,000 heart attacks a year could be prevented. I can only ask, how many more could be prevented if every workplace was a smoke-free zone? In the U.S., where this problem is being dealt with quite rigorously, the first statistics have been published. The best news is that no-smoking regulations enforced in several U.S. states have led to a drastic reduction in the total amount of cigarette sales. The tobacco industry will not be happy to hear it, but since laws banning smoking at work have been in effect, almost 10 billion (9.7 exactly, but why quibble?) fewer cigarettes have been smoked annually. This is almost 2% less than before the laws were in effect. Should the American government pass legislation banning smoking at the workplace throughout the U.S., which seems perfectly justified, then this number will more than double – to approximately 21 billion fewer cigarettes annually, a drop of 4.3%.

In Australia, smoking in public buildings is prohibited.

However, these figures do not reveal the number of smokers who have actually given up their habit completely. I think it is quite a few, because between 1990 and 1995, 12.5% fewer cigarettes were sold. This amounts to the astounding figure of 75.5 billion cigarettes.

In Australia cigarette smoking has been banned in public buildings since 1988. Over a seven-year observational period – during which private companies went along with the new regulation – cigarette sales went down a total of 7.7%. Respected scientists speculate that at least 25% of this drop can be attributed to the establishment of smoke-free zones.

Other Harmful Influences at Work

If I look back at my personal needs in the workplace, I must admit my greatest need was for silence. I know that there were and still are many colleagues who like to operate to the soft sounds of music. I, however, only wanted to be left in peace and quiet so that I could concentrate completely on the patient lying in front of me, something I felt I owed to that patient.

Nevertheless, I suffered considerably during my work for many years from an indirect effect which my workplace had on me. I came to hate the sound of my telephone ringing in the evenings once I was back home. I didn't sleep as well as I could have because I knew that each call meant bad news. Nobody phones a surgeon at three o'clock in the morning to let him know everything is OK.

Work can make us happy or ill. Three factors that can contribute to our not feeling well at work are:

1 passive smoking, as mentioned
2 dangerous environmental substances
3 the emotional situation (from boredom to frustration)

> *Check your workplace for possibly harmful substances. You spend a quarter of your life there!*

Perhaps you are exceedingly healthy, so being surrounded by things which cause illness doesn't affect you. But most of us are inside a body which cannot ward off every harmful influence. Dust mites, cat hair, mold, and the like are common allergens found indoors. They don't feature on your firm's salary list, but presumably they work harder than many of your co-workers. Only they don't work for you or with you, but against you.

If you're working year after year in the same environment you should take the time to have your surroundings checked for potentially dangerous substances. This includes substances that could be contained in furniture, rugs, or paint. They usually have impressive names like formaldehyde, pentachlorophenol, or pyrethroid and they can cause many different symptoms such as shortness of breath, irritated eyes, headaches, and nausea. If you are surrounded by them for years, even these comparatively harmless substances can lead to serious illness.

The worst of it is that you can do little against such substances other than change your job. In the history of the workplace it has not happened often that bosses have had the carpets in their underlings' offices removed just because someone thought that they were giving him headaches. Your only hope is to outmaneuvre your boss. Make him ill. No, not by attacking him. Just keep pointing out to him how dangerous such substances can be for him too. It often works wonders if you speak to him directly about cancer or a heart attack.

EMOTIONAL STRESSORS

In any case, don't think that your superior has a wonderful life just because his car is twice as big as yours. If you were to find out what problems he has, you would never want to change places with him. People who are in positions where they must often make very important decisions – deciding the fate of others – frequently take this to heart, to the point of having a higher risk of a heart attack. The Boston-based doctor Murray Mittleman questioned 791 people who had suffered a heart attack. Many had occupied positions in which they were responsible for hiring and firing.

> *More and more managers are bored with their work.*

The interesting aspect of the study proved to be that most of these people had their attack while under time pressures or psychological stress resulting from having to fire an employee. What was amazing in this study was that it confirmed that the number of patients suffering a cardiac arrest after being fired was fewer than among those who had to do the firing.

You won't believe it, but this is not the only health problem with which top managers are threatened. A much more serious danger facing us at the workplace is of an emotional nature. More and more firms, particularly in the U.S., are faced with the really tricky problem of boredom.

Some time ago several studies in the U.S. found that top executives change jobs because they have actually become bored with their work. This was very alarming news for business. Large concerns were, after all, investing millions in their leadership, keeping up their morale through such motivational schemes as seminars and feel-good weekends at fitness spas. All in vain? Motivational training seems to have no effect any more. More and more managers see no long-term sense in doing a particular job, and so they quit. *Burned Out at Work* is the title of a book written by Beverly Potter. This best-selling author mentions the time of year when this phenomenon most frequently occurs – in the "light" seasons of the year, spring and summer. During this period many people feel much more intensely that their lives are going nowhere and that they should be doing something more satisfying.

MONEY ISN'T EVERYTHING

Unbelievably it's not money any more that motivates employees. German psychologist Klaus Rempe specializes in work-related psychology and claims to have discovered in "at least 46%" of all

German employees the inner wish to quit their jobs. He maintains that there are various other factors why work today "tends to make people sick rather than give them joy." I think someone who enjoys his work will be able to accomplish things that are unimaginable to others. Rempe states, "Motivation is something only you can give yourself and that is the decisive factor." He lists the reasons for the current motivational crisis: lower performance initiative, rising expectations, yet at the same time a lack of identification with corporate goals, all this accompanied by a general lack of commitment.

Employers will not be able to combat this lingering problem by currying favours through incentives or other short-term solutions. It's important that they take on the role of the real "doer" and, in the best sense of the word, "entrepreneur." They need to demonstrate vision. As Rempe cleverly puts it, "People are not lazy, they just lack vision."

> *Most bosses lack vision.*

My Last Day

I would like to end this chapter with an example taken from my own life. It was a very important point for me, because it signaled the end of my surgical activities at the Groote Schuur Hospital in Cape Town. That was where I performed the first heart transplant on a human being in 1967. The end of my activities came six years before I would actually have had to retire, so it took everyone around me completely by surprise – except me. But I must admit that I took the decision to call it a day very suddenly indeed. It happened like this.

Members of the Faculty of Medicine of the University of Cape Town made a tour of the Medical School, visiting each department to find out what new equipment they required. They sat down in my office and, after a short introduction, asked me what my department was in urgent need of. My answer came without hesitation: A NEW HEAD.

When I was asked whether I was serious and why I had made this decision, I replied: "My work does not satisfy me anymore. In the morning I am not hungry for my job. It is time to quit and let a younger man take over."

That was the end of my professional career, and I must confess that I have never regretted that decision. Whenever someone has asked me for advice since then, I have told them: "If you wake up in the morning and you no longer look forward to your job, drop it and do something else." With all one's heart or not at all: that is a worthwhile motto for life.

Barnard Tips for a Healthy Heart
How to Pick the Right Company for You

1 Is the company's name-plate showy?
No problem, if the rest of it can compare. Otherwise, hands off: it could be more show than substance.

2 Are the carpets from the 1950s?
Retro-style is in fashion again, but 40-year-old coffee stains don't bode well.

3 Is the boss well dressed?
Don't judge too hastily. It may only be his wife's good taste, not his.

4 Is the boss badly dressed?
If he can't manage to keep himself in good shape, he probably can't manage to do it with the firm either.

5 Are your potential co-workers well dressed?
Usually a reliable sign that the firm pays more than minimum wage.

6 Is the receptionist snooty?
Careful: the boss might be chaotic. Could be a sign of creativity, but it might soon irritate you.

7 Are the business cards opulent?
Everyone wants to be the boss in that firm. That's only OK if you're a one (wo)man business.

8 Is the job offer generous?
If you are offered a higher wage than you would have asked for, take the job: this firm has vision.

9 Is the job offer bad?

Bad pay, lousy working conditions. If you take the job – where is your vision?

10 Do your friends work there?

Careful: the privately friendly might be vicious at work.

Work on Your Relationship

It's better not to tell your partner
absolutely everything – this strengthens
the relationship and your health.

I'm actually quite astounded at how little medical science has researched partnerships. One can find all sorts of studies on the healing process and on the health-damaging effects of our environment. But research studies that deal exclusively with the medical aspects of partnerships are still extremely rare. As I write this book I am going through another divorce. I would like to say only one thing about this. It is – once more – my fault that I did not try harder in our relationship to make things better. I don't want to say any more about my private life. One thing, however, is certain: I am going through very difficult times and I am in a very different state of mind from normal.

> *Marriage is the most important business in the world for me.*

You may find what I'm about to say a bit strange coming from me of all people. But marriage is for me the most important business in the world. And it is a business that must never be neglected; it needs constant attention. More so than in any other business – but the rewards resulting from this work are higher too.

The fact is that partnerships – and I mean well-balanced relationships between two people – can promote one's general feeling of well-being and positively influence one's health. One of the most serious threats to such a relationship is boredom. I know what I'm talking about here. Even in your "Good morning" and your "Good night," in the interest you show in clothing or the planning of a holiday, every spoken and unspoken communication with your partner should contain a little spark of creativity which gives new drive to that partnership. It's all contained in that not-so-old adage: variety is the spice of life.

The German psychologist Kurt Hahlweg warns that while the spring of a relationship brings with it the delightful question of who will be the first to undress, the autumn of a relationship is only too often signaled by the question: who will be the first to depart? Today every third marriage ends in divorce, with negative consequences for the health of all involved, man, woman, and children. Only the death of your beloved partner is more stressful than a divorce.

Keeping up a relationship means paying constant attention to it. This can contribute to your good health or it can – if based on subterfuge, for instance – make you ill. It has been shown that happily married people are less likely to die of a heart attack. One of the consequences of a divorce is an increased tendency to illness.

Every relationship has its crises. Money, education, sex – anything can be the subject of a dispute. Statistically speaking, marriages are most threatened after two, seven and twenty years. Why? Because people develop differently; because the couple may not have developed a system for coping with arguments, or they may have nothing to say to each other any more; because a new person has entered the scene; or because one of the partners feels that they are being taken for a ride and constantly treated as the dumb one in the relationship. Finally it might be because one partner wants to experience the fascination of a new relationship once more.

> *How can a relationship still be passionate when you know your partner inside out?*

Almost every relationship can be saved if a couple begin early enough. Practice prevention before all the dishes have been smashed:

- Talking is silver, silence is gold. Secrets are an essential factor in a relationship. "When partners know each other inside out," says psychologist Doris Wolf, "then that partnership lacks passion." An investigation by a German magazine revealed that what is most frequently kept secret are dreams about other men or women. Even extra-marital flings are admitted more often.

- Silence is silver, talking is gold. Not a contradiction but an addition. A good marriage is very much founded on the convention of good conversation. In moments of crisis this convention can take over the role of the fire department: the fire may spread up to a point – but no further. Any argument, no matter how serious or fundamental, must not be allowed to go beyond this limit. Otherwise the point will be reached, physically dangerous or otherwise, where neither can think of anything further to say. This point is where most marriages fail.

- Kissing is gold. The American psychologist Barbara de Angelis recommends: "Give your partner a kiss lasting at least 20 seconds at least once a day. This sets the energy flowing between the two of you."

- Praise is gold. The German psychologist Professor Kurt Hahlweg advises couples facing a crisis: "Look at your relationship like a savings account. One pays in and withdraws. Before one says something negative about one's partner, one has to praise him/her five times to build up sufficient credit to allow for the withdrawal."

- Cutting the umbilical cord is gold. Of course you are grateful to your parents for so much. But one can show one's gratitude in many ways. If your parents really love you, they will want you to do what brings you happiness and contributes to your good health. If you spend more time with your mother than with your wife, you should move back into your parents' house.

- Togetherness is gold. I know: you love to play golf but your wife doesn't much like to spend her time looking for little balls in the landscape. See to it that there are sufficient times of togetherness in your marriage. Create definite periods which are reserved for whole-family activities only.

- Sex is gold. The erotic has to be continually reinvented. Try to remain creative in the bedroom. If your partner keeps on discovering new sides of you during sex, he/she will feel less inclined to look elsewhere.

MARRIAGE CHECK: HOW GOOD IS YOUR RELATIONSHIP?

Do you and your partner stick together like glue? I have found a simple test in the *Berliner Kurier* newspaper which can tell you how your marriage is doing. If you answer "no" more often than "yes," you may be in trouble.

1 Do I still love him/her, or is it a relationship of convenience?
2 Do we like to sleep with each other?
3 Do we like to talk to each other?
4 Do I find pleasure in spoiling or surprising my partner?
5 Does my partner try to spoil or surprise me?
6 Do you still find it pleasant to listen to your partner?
7 Are you glad when he (she) is not there sometimes?
8 Do you still have common hobbies?
9 Do you often laugh together?
10 Have you ever been unfaithful to him/her?
11 Do you often argue and then take a long time to reconcile?
12 Does money throw a shadow over your relationship?
13 Does your marriage frequently turn into a power struggle?
14 Do you ever feel bored with your relationship?
15 Do you often squabble over your children?
16 Do you sometimes hate your partner (and find this more so of late)?
17 Do you dream of freedom without your partner?
18 Do you think your marriage could benefit from therapy?
19 Do you sometimes think: I've married too early?
20 Would you marry the same partner again?

Michael Lukas Moeller, a German psychologist at the medical faculty in Frankfurt, mentions one factor in relationships that can lead to illness: an inability to face conflict. I agree with this completely. My three marriages probably failed because I belong to this type. I don't like arguing. The better couples are able to communicate, the better and healthier their relationship.

But the number of couples able to do this is diminishing. "Till death us do part" is the way it's put in the Christian marriage ceremony. A Protestant parson from Germany once suggested that for safety's sake one might change this to "as long as possible."

25 Don't Give In to Your Mobile

Passive smoking can be dangerous.
But make sure that you don't breathe
in too much mobile phone "smog" either.

No epidemic in history has spread more quickly. Within a few years mobiles have been improved from clumsy, expensive, problem-prone objects into smart and handy lifestyle accessories. Mobiles are everywhere and they are becoming an ever greater nuisance. Whether we're enjoying a family meal, out driving or walking, at the theater, or on public transport, we stand a good chance of being disturbed by someone's mobile going off. Conversations of more than two sentences are scarcely possible because they get nipped in the bud by a mobile call. "Yes, well, where were we?" has become a very popular question.

Passive smoking is one thing, but what should we call the way mobiles invade our private lives even without our actually owning one? Passive phoning? Perhaps. In any case, I think that this theme will become a topic of extensive discussion and research in the next few years. Because mobiles are not only multiplying fast, they are becoming increasingly shameless, intruding everywhere they can be carried – and I mean everywhere! Mobiles have entered the bedroom, the children's room, the vacation. The frightening possibility that we could miss out on something makes us slaves to technology.

I am not against the mobile as such. I have already mentioned that I obtained a mobile because it is a practical thing to have. But we have to set limits, not only for ourselves but for others as well. Mobiles irritate more people than one might believe. A few years ago one could smile about restaurants that prohibited the use of mobiles on their premises. It's quite possible that we will soon see something similar to the ruling governing smoking being instituted in many public places – a separation of spaces for use by mobile users and non-mobile users.

> *Can something which inhibits safety on board a plane really be no threat to your health?*

It has not – yet – been shown that mobiles can inflict physical damage, but I think that they simply cannot be good for your health. How could something be completely safe for us which has to be turned off on board a plane because it can interfere with the navigational instrumentation? What we already know is that people using cardiac pacemakers have to keep mobiles at a defined distance away from themselves. A mobile with an output of 0.6 watts must be kept at least 6 inches away from your pacemaker. Mobiles with an output of three watts or more must be kept at least 12 inches away. Always use your mobile with the ear on the opposite side of your pacemaker.

What even healthy people should take to heart as well is the following advice: whether it's switched on or off, don't carry your mobile in your breast pocket or – very popular – on your belt like a revolver. Since the subject is still new there are, of course, no long-term studies available yet. But there are concerns by doctors and scientists that should be taken seriously, and I dare to say that sometime in the not so distant future we will be unpleasantly surprised to learn about the negative effects of the cellular boom.

I readily admit that mobiles bother me. I find it inconsiderate to make a phone call in front of other people and it's plainly disrespectful. But mobiles are status symbols. When I used to go to parties in the U.S. people would come to me and proudly show me their bypass operation scars. Now they get out their mobiles and try to tell me about the advantages of these new companions. They soon notice how disinterested I am.

I have split mobile owners into two groups:

1 the "Talkers"
2 the "Walkers."

The "Talkers" get on our nerves by surrounding themselves with a pretentious aura of importance, gesticulating wildly, and talking loudly. Their presence used to be most obvious in public places frequented by the better-off, such as restaurants, airports, and conference centers. With the proliferation of mobiles they are, however, increasingly becoming a feature of public spaces in general.

The "Walkers" are always on the go. They telephone as they walk along the street and even while crossing it. They create the impression that they have to dash from one appointment to the next – very active, indispensable cogs in the wheels of society. They don't irritate me so much any more; I increasingly find myself feeling sorry for them.

> *When my wife's mobile broke down, I "used" it all over Cape Town.*

To prevent any problems with mobiles for myself I used one as a joke some years ago. It was my wife's phone, a wonderful looking device that one day just stopped working. So I took it and carried it around with me. It served me well. If a conversation or company bored me I took it out, went to a quiet corner and pretended to talk on the phone. On the busy streets of Cape Town I sometimes got out my mobile and pretended to be answering someone's call. I admit that it was sometimes fun to do this. "That Barnard," people would say, "is still with it technologically." Sometimes people asked me for my number, but I only gave it on the rarest occasions. Of course it had no value whatsoever. No one could reach me under the number I gave out anyway, but it did raise my social status to be the proud owner of a mobile phone unreachable for virtually everyone – actually everyone. But some could at least say they'd tried to reach me.

Know When to Quit

The daily office battle may leave you
with only two courses of action:
you fight or you quit.

The fight for jobs, the fight for a higher social status is getting tougher – at least in the so-called "civilized" Western world. New technologies and values – obsession with youth and venture capitalism are but two illustrations of this – have only accelerated this development. To be brilliant at one's job today doesn't necessarily require specialized knowledge, more important are the elbows needed to clear the way to the top.

In the early 1950s I once felt very threatened in my development and my prospects for the future. That was in Cape Town on one specific occasion when I was still an assistant to Professor Jan Louw. During an operation he found fault with everything I did. Here I was too slow, there I wasn't attentive enough. In a word, I felt absolutely miserable. That was when I decided on the following action: I slowly stepped back from the operating table and just as slowly pulled off my gloves and left the operating theatre. When I happened to meet Professor Louw the next day, he merely said to me, "Don't you think you owe me an apology?" And I replied: "On the contrary, I am hoping for an apology from you."

Work satisfies us or it makes us ill. For more and more people their work is becoming a burden which overtaxes them physically and psychologically. Strange: for hundreds of years men and women suffered the burden of hard manual labour. Now that they

158

are housed in pleasantly furnished offices, they become a burden to one another. Are our jobs so undemanding that we must take it out on our colleagues?

Conflict Costs

Over 6% of the total population have at one time or another become the victims of conflict at work. In Germany that amounts to nearly 1 million people; in the U.S. it would be around 5 million. According to psychologists, bullying in the workplace costs industry billions annually. People who are harassed, yelled at, or threatened by their colleagues and their superiors show less enthusiasm, take more sick leave, and retire earlier.

Bullying can be very low key at the outset. At first colleagues don't ask you any more whether you would like to go to the cafeteria with them. Then important information is withheld from you. Suddenly data disappears from your computer, or you are deliberately confronted with a no-win situation. "Oh, sorry, I quite forgot to tell you, the boss would like you to prepare a 100-page concept on our new product by tomorrow." The last stage is the use of physical force.

When bullying takes place in an office, superiors play a decisive role. They choose sides in conflict situations and in this way they direct the action. Increasingly, superiors are themselves initiating bullying attacks. Anyone wanting to get rid of an awkward colleague in a way not detrimental to himself, begins to try and make that person unhappy at work. Experts estimate that in three-quarters of all attempts at harassment, the immediate superior has played some role.

Harassment or bullying takes place with men and women, but women react to it differently than men. Women more frequently look to themselves as having provoked the attack in some way or other, and they don't defend themselves as forcefully. Men tend to go on the offensive more often and to seek legal aid.

The physical consequences are the same for men and women. At first it manifests itself through seemingly harmless symptoms such as migraine or abdominal pain. Then the body reacts with sleeplessness. Finally, psychosomatic ailments make their appearance.

These can range from asthma to problems of the cardiovascular system. And social contacts usually dry up. The person tends to withdraw more and more into his own world because he perceives the world around him as hostile.

Sick Building Syndrome

It's interesting to note in this context that the German University of Jena, after a five-year study, was apparently able to broaden the description of what is known as "Sick Building Syndrome." This term was originally used to describe illnesses which could be caused by harmful materials situated in the workplace. The Jena scientists were able to establish that not only is the physical environment responsible for psychological and health problems, but the general working climate as well. Using a rather remarkable 5,000 people as a test group (in 14 different buildings at 1,500 different workplaces), the researchers found evidence that headaches, fatigue, and even mucous membrane infections could be traced back to people feeling mentally uncomfortable in their working environment. This was independent of other factors such as building materials, bad ventilation, or other hazardous substances in the working environment. Professor Wolfgang Bischof, leader of the research study, summarized the results as follows: "Specific measures taken to improve the atmosphere at work are often more important than proper operation of the air-conditioning."

Bullying is not so often practiced on the lazy and ineffectual colleagues in an office, but rather on the diligent and more talented. These quick, able, and committed workers are an irritation to those around them because they offer superiors a standard of work against which performance is measured and with which colleagues have to compete. There are classic risk groups: doctors are seven times as likely to be bullied at the workplace, teachers three times as likely, and public service employees one-and-a-half times as likely to be at risk of such treatment.

An advice center was established in Berlin in the mid-1990s devoted to helping the victims of harassment. "Solution" (*Wirkstoff*) tries to help people deliberately discriminated against in the workplace. In its first year the following trends emerged:

- About 40% of the people who came to the center worked in the public service sector.
- More than a quarter of the victims of bullying had already been made ill by their problems at work.
- Two-thirds spoke about having psychosomatic problems.
- Some 5% felt they had been sexually harassed in their workplace.

> *When your job begins to stink – quit!*

The victim of a bullying attack can do little about it. It seems to be of little use talking to colleagues about it. Fear of dismissal, fear of being transferred elsewhere, envy, jealousy – many factors can contribute to bullying behavior. In such a climate it is important that you try as far as possible to keep a clear head. Do your own analysis, considering all the facts, and then decide: are your colleagues' attacks so bad that they cause you serious physical and/or emotional suffering? Do the problems at work interfere negatively with your private life? And just as important: do you think that things are going to get worse rather than better? If this is what you feel, then you probably owe it to yourself to look for another job and prepare to tender your resignation.

27 Let the Sun Shine In

Cooler temperatures raise the risk
to your heart. When it gets cold the
rate of heart attacks rises.

I think that things are sometimes simpler than they seem to us. In Chapter 7 I told you some of the secrets of the Crete diet. The people on that Greek island suffer fewer heart attacks than anyone else in the civilized world. In the last few years researchers have explained the low rate of heart attacks particularly in terms of the islanders' healthy eating habits. A lot of vegetables, little meat, some wine; I think this explanation is not comprehensive enough, though, because I have the impression that the secret lies at least in part in the climate. People living in southern climes have more access to sunlight, hence they have "lighter" hearts.

That may at first sound a little paradoxical, but it's really true. Whether our heart is sound also depends to a certain degree on the time of year. Two researchers proved this independently of each other: Professor Robert A. Kloner from Los Angeles and Sandrine Danet from Lille, France.

The European study was the first one that established a direct connection between meteorology and the myocardiac death rate. The researchers found that when outside temperatures sank by 10 degrees or more, the heart attack rate rose by approximately 13%. The French researchers also studied the effect of variations of air pressure. The result: a 10-millibar difference – regardless of whether it was up or down – increased the heart attack rate between 11% and 12%.

> *When the temperature sinks, the risk of heart attack rises by 13%.*

Among the 3,330 people included in the study were those who had never before experienced heart problems. Among people who had previously had a heart attack and among older people the risk rate was even higher. The time span of the study, which for the first time provided conclusive evidence of the interaction between weather and myocardiac frequency, was particularly impressive. Sandrine Danet and her colleagues worked a total of 10 years. Their research formed a part of the World Health Organisation's MONICA project, an undertaking that has in the last few years come to be considered internationally authoritative in the field of research into heart disease.

The conclusion reached? The colder the season, the more heart attacks. It's interesting to note that in his study in Los Angeles Professor Kloner came to the same conclusion. Kloner also registered the most coronary deaths in winter months, over a 10-year time span. In the months of July, August and September the heart attack rate in the study group fell by 25%.

The fact that the Californian climate does not, for the most part, have extreme temperature fluctuations means that the two pieces of research were undertaken under very different climatic circumstances. This lends further validity to the findings. It's possible to view our instinctive reaction to increase our calcium and nutritional intake during the winter months – to help us cope with climatic change – as a possible trigger for the coronary problems incurred. The other possible explanation: the greater risk of viral infections during the winter months could also lead to the rise in the cardiac problems.

> *The nicest sun is the one that shines on your house.*

One should avoid making hasty judgments. Of course it's better for the heart if it isn't exposed to great temperature variations.

But before you pack your bags and hasten southwards: the best sun is still the one shining on your house, even if it is sometimes not as warm as you'd like.

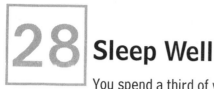

28 Sleep Well

You spend a third of your life in the bedroom. Make more of it than a wardrobe.

You are a workhorse and spend most of your time in the office? You're a real family man and the living room at home is where you hang out? All well and good. But don't forget that another room plays a most important role in your life: your bedroom. That's where you spend a third of your life. And if your relationship is healthy, you also experience some of your happiest moments in this room. Perhaps it's time to give some thought to how you should arrange the most important room in your life.

> *Keep your bedroom arrangements simple. You can show off your possessions somewhere else.*

I call them the "fab four," taking the term from the Beatles. Four things are of importance for me in a bedroom:

1   no television
2   no computer
3   no animals
4   always clean sheets.

I am not afraid of electric currents, but I simply don't like electronic gadgets in rooms meant for resting. They bring hustle and bustle into our lives, just what we want to avoid when resting. Computers remind us of work. Even if you love your job – not in the bedroom! Keep your work and your private life apart. After all, you don't go on holiday with your boss, do you? And there are other things you can do without in your bedroom:

- the wrong mattress
  When you have made your bed, you will have to lie on it. Your car has leather seat covers, but at home you're still using the mattress your mother-in-law gave you at your wedding? Treat yourself to something new. Something that has to support your weight every night can't last for ever. A first-hand test is necessary and the rule of thumb here is simple as well: light-weights should always take a soft mattress and heavyweights a hard one.
- too much opulence
  A bedroom should be kept simple. There is no need for much more than a bed, a cupboard and space to change clothes, even if you could easily afford more. This will leave you in every sense with room to breathe. You can show off your wealth in other places.
- the wrong attitude
  Keep boredom out of the bedroom. Try to remain sexually creative throughout your life. To give is more enriching than to receive.
- the wrong nourishment
  Most of us eat our main meal of the day in the evening. This need not be a bad thing, unless you then go straight to bed. As a rule the last meal should be taken at least three hours before bedtime. A glass of good red wine will help you to relax.

> *Sport before going to bed is not a good idea. In the evening your body is programmed for rest.*

- the wrong rituals
  Exquisitely scented oils are OK in the bedroom as long as the vapors don't take your breath away. But taking a sauna just before lying down is not a good idea at all. You should have

completed that relaxation of the muscles and the senses at least two hours before going to bed – to then sleep like a baby.

- the wrong sport

  Of course you should be active – but at the right time. Sport in the morning is good, but it doesn't suit everyone. Sport in the evening is less good because you should be programming your body for rest. Four hours should elapse between fitness training and going to bed.

- the wrong colors

  Sleep in a sparsely furnished, well-ventilated room and be sure to take the colors of your surroundings into consideration. Wood and earth tones should be a priority because these help to instil a soothing ambience.

Colors and people – in the last few years a science of its own has been developed out of this combination. It is based on the assumption that colors play a bigger role in our lives than is generally believed. Very revealing, it seems to me, is what color psychologists can deduce from our cars.

- If you buy a red car, you want to show that you have an inclination towards speed and the erotic.
- Blue cars signal steadiness and sobriety.
- Yellow reveals a sunny nature.
- Drivers of grey cars always want to do things correctly.
- Black cars are not only the prerogative of statesmen.
- Drivers of white cars prefer to go unnoticed.

29 Keep a Pet

Dogs are, after all, only human.
So they deserve a medal for what
they do for us.

Approximately 10% of the people in the U.K. with cats or dogs for pets are over 60 years old. Studies have confirmed that people who have animals in their homes have less of a tendency to acquire heart and circulatory problems, are less lonely, and make social contacts more easily than those without pets. Animals help us get rid of aggression towards others, they get us to relax and think of other things.

I know what I'm talking about. After all, I bought an animal farm in the vicinity of Cape Town in South Africa. It consists largely of animals that are in danger of extinction, such as some zebra and antelope species, which I hope I can save for my grandchildren. But I must say that just looking at these wonderful animals gives me a sense of serenity.

> *My pets: two rhinos, zebras, antelopes. But I really love scorpions.*

When I was a child we always had pets at home, but I didn't like dogs. How different my attitude to dogs is today – I'll come to this later. As a boy I loved three kinds of animals: bantam chickens, cats – and scorpions. I don't know what attracted me to these dangerous creatures. They could be found under every stone in our neighborhood. Baboons love to eat them, but I never tried one.

168

Today I love one animal more than all the others: the dog. An animal that I never took much notice of previously, we would do well to erect a monument to this faithful friend. Its unbelievable, unconditional faithfulness always moves me. I know that for my dog I will always be a miserable scoundrel because before we did the first human transplants, we experimented with dogs, but what other choice did we have?

I often took this matter to heart, particularly because my first wife – who loved dogs – and I later brought home two special examples. Out of pity we accepted Sixpence, a mongrel, from the laboratory; Ringo was a gift from a patient. From beginning to end it was an extraordinary experience in faithfulness, loyalty, and affection which we were given in return for their daily meal. Strange: Sixpence only survived our divorce by a few days. My ex-wife buried him in the yard and even placed a cross on the fresh soil. Two weeks later she found Ringo dead next to the grave. I think he died of a broken heart.

> *Children who have pets are more diligent and balanced; they are also happier.*

Animals deserve our respect; they are our soul mates. In Berlin there is an organization called Life with Animals. For more than 10 years they have established so-called petting zoos in hospitals. Volunteers take care of the animals – goats, sheep, dogs – while the patients can enjoy their presence and profit from it. According to Maoris Huff, a member of Life with Animals who has many years of experience, "The success has been surprising. Even patients with severe illnesses, including those suffering from heart disease, benefit from the presence of the animals and from being able to stroke them."

In the United States this form of "therapy" is known and recognized. This so-called "Dog-day visitation" is part of a social therapy program offered in nursing homes where keeping animals is otherwise not wanted or even allowed.

Animals Make Children Happy

Seldom do children ask for anything so adamantly as for a pet. The result: the completely unnerved parents usually give in to the pleadings of the child. I wonder if many of them would be more willing to give in if they were aware of the statistics? Some 95% (!) of all pet owners report that their pet has had a positive influence on their child's development. The other positive aspects are also quite impressive:

- Children with pets have an increased sense of duty (93% of pet owners reported this).
- They have an increased sense of responsibility (95%).
- They demonstrate increased solicitousness (91%), and are generally more attentive.
- They have an increased sense of the natural world (81%).
- They seem to get more joy out of life (68%).
- Their characters seem more balanced, more well adjusted (58%).

A relevant study at the University of Montreal showed an increase in intelligence and fewer bouts of depression among pet owners.

Winston Churchill's mocking words on this theme seem misanthropic rather than anti-animal: "I don't like cats. They seem too proud, always looking down their noses at me. I don't like dogs either. Their downcast look makes them seem too servile. What I really like are pigs. Why? They consider themselves equal to man." Perhaps he had a point.

30 | Let There Be Light

The best medicine for depression
and heaviness of heart: go into the sun.

Were the famous last words of Germany's greatest poet and writer, Johann Wolfgang von Goethe, really "More light" ("Mehr Licht")? Or did he say, "No more" ("Mehr nicht")? If the "More light" theory is true, this would confirm at least two further theories. The first is the story about how difficult it was for this acclaimed genius to leave this life. I once heard that he screamed for a week in fear anticipating his impending death before, completely exhausted, he finally sank back into his bed and died. While the words "more light" would fit well with this version of Goethe's final moments, they would even better suit the stories that we have heard from people who have had "near-death" experiences. The Swiss researcher Kübler-Ross has written up many such experiences. Their stories always have one thing in common: they describe travelling down a long dark tunnel which they are pulled out of at the last moment. A long dark tunnel and Goethe's call for more light? That fits.

I too have had some experience in this sphere and have helped to bring people who were already dying back to life. On occasion when we would resuscitate patients whose hearts had stopped, using massage or electro-shock treatment, they would recount similar impressions. They also kept on about a bright light at the end of the long dark tunnel – like a ray of hope.

I believe that this light phenomenon can be traced back to a natural, biochemical process in the brain. I believe it is the result of an acute lack of oxygen brought about by insufficient blood flow.

Death holds many mysteries, however. One tragic death that really shocked me was Princess Diana's. I had been an ardent admirer of hers. It still gives me great pleasure today to know that I was reasonably well acquainted with her. Just two months before her death she had invited me to a private dinner at Kensington Palace. I still honor the present she gave me on that occasion, and I wear it only on special occasions – a dark blue silk tie with an African pattern.

Her death stunned me all the more as I was able to get a look at the particulars of the autopsy findings very soon after her death. I don't want to make a big "what if" and "if only" out of this. But I also don't want to keep quiet here. I think she could have been saved, because according to the report which I have seen, she died of internal bleeding. The injury which caused the bleeding was to a vein which doesn't bleed particularly quickly, in fact it bleeds rather slowly. What I want to say here is that if Princess Diana had been brought to hospital within 10 minutes of the accident – something which should easily have been possible – and, once there, had been cared for properly, she could have survived.

Let There Be Light

There is hardly a more significant energy source than light in its influence on every human action. We know that lack of light creates fear and that "hot light" fosters aggression. When the weather acts crazy and for days there is cloud cover without even a glimpse of sun, it's not only sensitive souls who react with a somewhat subdued disposition.

Scientific research has confirmed that light affects our state of mind immensely. Besides our psyche, it also affects our bodies. Light also has a kind of healing quality. It is now being used to combat one of the increasing problems of our time, depression. In my case, I always felt worse after a difficult and very mentally draining operation if it was raining or the sky was filled with clouds. Sunshine was a big help.

So the sun usually has a literally heart-warming effect on me.

Activity

31 Start Now

You can reach the ripe old age of 120 and even more. Every hour of fast walking increases your life span by 60 minutes.

After my fourth son was born, my wife Karin said to me: "Chris, it's time for you to do something for your fitness again. I can't push a pram *and* a wheelchair."

Actually it was true I had become somewhat "rusty" over previous years. In South Africa I have a life-long membership in a fitness club, but I hadn't been there for quite a while. Due to my travels it is difficult for me to participate in my favorite sports and hobbies, like fishing and hunting. This is even though sport has played an important role in my life. During my school days I was captain of my rugby team, and in tennis I once even became school champion. I was also a passable swimmer.

> *Why I played rugby, how I became a tennis champ. And why I gave it all up.*

But then I went to university and everything changed. I was terribly afraid of failing my courses. My father was a poor man who had to save all he could to send his children to university. I still vividly recall the time my elder brother failed an exam. He was so ashamed that he didn't come out of his room for two days.

That left a deep impression on me. When I entered university I first gave up women and then, a short time later, sport as well.

175

Why play sport or take exercise? For hundreds of years people seemed to do all right without fitness studios and roller blades. Winston Churchill hated sport and lived to be 91. Millions injure themselves in some form of sporting activity every year. Nothing proves that more active people get more out of life.

There are also dozens of classic sports ailments that can make life difficult for you. Anything from muscle aches to meniscus problems.

In Germany alone, the treatment of injuries costs over 27 billion marks every year. A large proportion of these injuries are the result of sporting accidents.

So why exercise? Because there is no other way which can so easily lengthen our life expectancy. Sport is also the only way I know of for making us younger – in body and in spirit.

1 Sport is healthy.
  Sport and exercise help the body in its battle against many illnesses: cancer, arthritis, osteoporosis, migraine, asthma, and stroke.
2 Sport makes you happy.
  Exercise activates the body to produce endorphins, the so-called "happiness hormones."
3 Sport promotes a sense of achievement.
  Keeping fit is an achievement. The soul also benefits from this sense of accomplishment.
4 Sport keeps you trim.
  No diet plan can so effectively get rid of excess pounds.
5 Sport helps reduce debt.
  The cost of treating sport-related injuries and poor health brought on by a lack of exercise means that health services around the world are running at a deficit.
6 Sport increases your life expectancy.
  Walking to work can reduce the chance of dying from a heart or circulatory ailment by half. Every hour spent walking fast will extend your life by 60 minutes.
7 Sport stimulates the body's defences.
  Exercise can help to prevent colds. Researchers at an American university also found out that athletes produce more "good" cytocines: proteins which can inhibit arteriosclerosis.

8 Sport helps combat sleeplessness.
   Researchers at the University of Arizona discovered that people who walk a couple of miles every day reduce their risk of sleeping poorly by a third.

9 Sport helps you get rid of worries.
   After looking at the results of several studies, the American scientific journal *The Physician and Sport-Medicine* came to the conclusion that participating in a sport can help prevent depression.

10 Sport keeps you alert.
   Two psychiatrists writing in the *British Medical Journal* were able to verify that measured endurance training can help reduce the occurrence of exhaustion.

11 Sport keeps you young.
   Exercise can help slow the muscle deterioration associated with aging. A recent U.S. study found that a 70-year-old exercising regularly over six months could have the same lung capacity as a 50-year-old.

12 Sport can help beat stress.
   A person with more muscle can reduce the level of stress hormones in the body more quickly.

Above all, sport and exercise are true miracle workers for the heart. Exercising reduces blood pressure and cholesterol levels, minimizes the possibility of weight gain, and can protect against diabetes – four of the main risk factors for heart and circulatory diseases.

There is a great deal of evidence to support the fact that exercise is good for the heart. One of the most important studies was conducted on 10,269 graduates of the renowned Harvard University who were observed over an 8-year time span. The group who took part in two to three hours of endurance training per week had the best results. These graduates were found to have 60% less risk of dying from heart-related illnesses.

Sport can lower your risk of heart attack by up to 72%. Even smokers can benefit.

The Finnish sports physician Timo A. Laaka came up with similar findings in his study of men between the ages of 42 and 60. Men who spent about two hours a week on fitness training reduced their heart attack risk by 72%.

Sport and exercise even show a positive effect on smokers who cannot quit their habit. Researchers at the University of Malmö in Sweden established that smokers who participated in a fitness program had a 40% less heart attack risk than sedentary puffers.

The positive effects of sport on health can, however, be partially ruined by passive smoke inhalation. Doctors at the University of Freiburg (Germany) were able to prove that physically fit men clearly have more elastic arteries than their lazier brethren. However, if these same men were subjected to cigarette smoke the elasticity of the arteries was reduced by 20% within five minutes.

If we know that exercise is good for us, then why do so few of us actually exercise?

Many initially manage to conquer their weaker selves, only to quit again after a short period of time. More than half of all those who start exercising quit after six weeks.

I think there is a simple reason why so many are exercise-shy: they choose a sport that doesn't suit them and which gives them no pleasure.

Participating in sport must be fun and never boring. I have always chosen to engage in sports that provide me with a challenge. However, exercising can be very simple. While I was a student I didn't have very much money, so I walked to and from university – about three miles – every day. Today we know that walking can lengthen one's life. Perhaps the lack of money in my youth has helped me to live a long life!

> *When I was a student I always walked to and from university. Perhaps that is why I am still alive at my age.*

It's good to experiment with exercising. If you are interested in trying a new kind of sport or a new fitness concept you should try it – even if you are older. Exercising helps to keep you mentally fit, presents you with challenges, perhaps even conveys a sense of achievement, and helps you to meet new people.

However it is important for you not to overestimate your body or your abilities. Only you can determine what form of exercise is best for you. Only a sport that you have fun at will keep you consistently active.

Choose your ideal sport by using the following four criteria:

1 It has to suit you. Don't force yourself to participate in a sport just because it's trendy.
2 It must be fun. Only if you have fun at what you do will you do it regularly.
3 It must suit your physical abilities and condition. For every physical type there is an ideal sport.
4 It must present a challenge. Sport should always provide competition – be it against yourself or others.

The American fitness magazine *Men's Health* recently tried to assist its readers in selecting a sport best suited to them. The process was split into body types:

Body Type	Short, thin legs
Role Model	Andre Agassi
Ideal Sports	Tennis, riding, bicycling, running, endurance training
Advantages	Minimal body weight, therefore reduced need for calories, efficient calorie burning

Body Type	Short, muscular
Role Model	Pele
Ideal Sports	Football, gymnastics, karate, ice hockey, mountain climbing, skiing (slalom), squash
Advantages	Excellent sense of balance, good mobility, perfect harmony between size and strength, good reflexes

Body Type	Stocky, very muscular, short, thick-limbed
Role Model	Mike Tyson
Ideal Sports	Wrestling, weight-lifting, boxing, rugby
Advantages	Low center of balance makes it hard to lose it

Short limbs provide perfect leverage and excellent power

> *Do what Andre Agassi and Mike Tyson did – choose a sport that suits you.*

Body Type	Medium size/light (body like Pele only 8 inches taller)
Role Model	Steve Redgrave (Olympic rowing champion)
Ideal Sports	Swimming, rowing, diving, baseball, cricket, skiing (giant slalom)
Advantages	Too gangly for power sports. Ideal for steady, continual distribution of strength as in swimming

Body Type	Tall, thin, muscular
Role Model	Michael Jordan
Ideal Sports	Tennis, volleyball, golf, basketball, cricket
Advantages	Long arms with little muscle but great speed have good leverage (particularly useful for tennis)

Body Type	Tall, muscular
Role Model	Herman Mayer
Ideal Sports	Weight-lifting, basketball, sailing, skiing (downhill)
Advantages	Good combination of size and strength. Good leverage

There are, of course, many other kinds of sports besides those mentioned above which can be enjoyed by all body types until late in life. These include the classic "heart sports" such as walking (fast-paced), swimming, cross-country running, cycling and hiking.

> *The simplest sport: walk to work and back again.*

We can find the simplest methods of keeping fit everywhere around us. Don't use the elevator but take the stairs to get to your office. Park your car as far away as possible from the entrance to the shopping mall. Walk home from work every now and then. Maybe you will live to 120 or even older.

32 Be a Winner

Every sport is a competition.

You decide if you belong to

the winners or the losers.

A few years ago I was visiting Tyrol (Austria) and happened to meet Niki Lauda, the famous Formula One champion. I am not very good at alpine skiing so I decided to go cross-country skiing instead. Niki Lauda, however, indulged in so many sports activities during our time there that my muscles ached just watching him. When I got a chance to talk to him I told him that I was astonished that a racing car driver had to train so much considering that all he had to do in his sport was sit down and drive. Later I realized why he trained so hard. It was the year he became Formula One world champion again.

I mention this anecdote because for me sport and success represent an inseparable combination. I don't know anyone who loses continually and still enjoys participating in his or her sport. I want to show you how everyone can become a champion.

Exercise is like sex: it is a basic need. You don't have to give your body any signals – it will automatically announce its desire for movement in one way or another.

It's important to know that we have a natural inclination for exercise even though this feeling varies from person to person. For some it's enough to take a walk or do some gardening. Others experience a kind of euphoria upon completing a marathon.

> *If you always lose at sport, you will lose your enthusiasm and enjoyment in the activity.*

Why do some people enjoy sport and others not? I think the answer is quite simple: because some always lose and others always win. But it doesn't have to be this way.

Remind yourself of how you first came into contact with sport: as children we play football in the park, baseball or hockey out in the road, and perhaps volleyball or track and field events at school. Each competition divided the participants into two groups: the winners and the losers.

Those who could kick a ball further and harder, those who could run faster, took a positive picture of sport with them into adulthood. For many others sport became associated with feelings of frustration and failure.

However, sport does not always have to have winners and losers. If everyone chooses a sport that can make them champion, then they will be successful. Victory does not always mean being first or fastest. Success can also mean having the willpower to finish running a race, or to reach the finish line in a cycling event.

Therefore, for me, good sports have two rules:

1 They have to make you a winner. If you're always on the losing end at football or tennis, then find success in jogging, swimming, or cycling.
2 It has to challenge you. Sport is competitive. Either battle yourself or others.

> *In sport the first half-hour is the most important for your body.*

But how much competition is healthy? The wonderful thing about exercise is that it works from the very first moment. Two years ago the American epidemiologist Claudia Chae from Brigham and Women's Hospital in Boston concluded that exercise creates a positive effect within minutes. If someone regularly works out he or she does not have to do it for hours on end. The first half-hour is decisive. The American Heart Association, the largest American health organization, came to the same conclusion and offers the following recommendations:

- Exercise at least three times a week.
- The exercises should last between 30 minutes and 1 hour.
- It is wise to spread out your exercise time schedule over the week.

The renowned American Centers for Disease Control and the Organization of American Sports Physicians recommend:

- Thirty minutes of moderate exercise every day.
- Burn 200 calories a day through some form of exercise. This can be achieved through one hour of gardening.
- Start today. The first 25 minutes are the most effective.

If you want to start doing sport later in life, consult a doctor before you begin.

The most important rule, however, is: if you are over 40 years old and have never really exercised then it is advisable before you start a training program to first see a doctor. He or she can ascertain just how much exercise your heart can take. Remember: you could have a heart problem without knowing it and without it affecting your daily life. But as soon as you start with sport or exercise, this problem could become life-threatening.

Don't expect miracles from exercising. Only if your lifestyle changes over a period of time and you exercise regularly will your body respond noticeably and appropriately. A study undertaken at the University of Emory in Atlanta confirms this. Students who took part in a short-lived physical fitness program had worse cholesterol levels than students who did not exercise at all.

However, before you go back to your couch, take the following into consideration: students who exercised for two years had by far the best levels.

Barnard Tips for a Healthy Heart
The Ten Best Tips for Enjoying Sport

1 **Become a champion.**
Find a sport in which you can continually break your own "personal best" or can beat others.

2 **Save time.**
Ninety minutes a week is fine to start off with. Watch less television.

3 **Have fun.**
If you force yourself to exercise, you will quickly lose interest.

4 **Set yourself a goal.**
Don't be off and running without a plan. Only a well-conceived and well-organized exercise programme will lead to success.

5 **Do it regularly.**
Make exercise part of your daily routine, like brushing your teeth.

6 **Concentrate.**
Don't read the newspaper while exercising. Sport deserves your full attention.

7 **Take time off.**
If you're not in the mood for exercising then don't force yourself to do it.

8 **Warm up.**
It's just like sex: you wouldn't want to forego foreplay, would you?

9 **Don't over-exercise.**
If your pulse is above normal levels for a long time after you've finished exercising, you're overdoing it. Increase your activity levels slowly over a long time.

10 **Think long term.**
Endurance training burns more fat than short intense spurts of exercise.

33 Phone Your Way to Fitness

Do keep-fit exercises in your office
every two hours. A simple tennis ball
can assist in relieving tension.

We all have become somewhat sedentary. We sit in the office, in our free time, and even when we go on holiday. The consequences are becoming increasingly – and painfully – obvious: red and burning eyes, headaches, and muscle tension. A survey of 2,000 office workers revealed that 30% suffered from fatigue, sleep disorders, and concentration lapses. Two-thirds complained about back and limb pain.

Computer work is causing an increasing number of illnesses. Many physicians recommend that no one should work more than five hours a day in front of a computer screen. But almost a third of all office workers spend more than this recommended time in front of their monitors. Those who spend the most time in front of a computer suffer double the amount of eye problems as those who keep to the recommended hours.

The World Heath Organization (WHO) presented the so-called "Ottawa Charter" more than 12 years ago: "The way and form in which a society organizes work, and working and recreational conditions should be a source of health and not a cause of illnesses."

The status quo looks different. A new study commissioned by the German State Institute for Work Protection and Work Medicine (Bundesanstalt für Arbeitsschutz und Arbeitsmedizin) came to the following conclusion: if more than half of a person's time at work is spent in front of a computer screen, the health risks rise considerably. Already two-thirds of all employees complain of back pain. Almost half suffer from headaches, and approximately 40% complain about eye problems.

As our body finds it more and more difficult to cope with the demands of daily living, we fall ill more often. Backache in particular has become a widespread malady. Every fifth worker's reason for staying at home is given as problems associated with the spinal column. Also on the increase: a survey carried out by Germany's medical aid societies found that 8% cite a heart problem as the reason for staying away from work.

One of the biggest problems of modern working conditions is that we don't grant our body a reprieve. But working in front of a computer screen practically demands a break – so that we can recover from the strain on our eyes and to relieve the tension in our back. Breaks also benefit employers because they definitely increase the workforce's performance abilities.

> *A Swedish doctor has developed the best training program for the office.*

In Part II of this book I have already mentioned a few methods of relieving stress at the office. Now I would like to give you a few more simple keep-fit exercises that can be done at virtually every workstation. You should do some of these simple exercises every two hours.

Muscle Relaxation in the Office

Edmund Jacobson, a doctor from Sweden who emigrated to the United States at the beginning of the 20th century, developed the most renowned exercises for relaxing the muscles. Jacobson worked at Harvard University where he developed the so-called Progressive Muscle Tension Relief method. The basic idea for the exercises is as simple as it is clever: Jacobson discovered that muscles can best be relieved of stress if they are first flexed and then abruptly released.

Today Progressive Muscle Tension Relief has many different variations. I would like to give you a few examples of how to use this method during the day at work. The exercises can be done lying down, sitting, or standing. In what follows I want to restrict myself to exercises to be done standing up. Because most of us have "sitting" jobs it is a good idea to stand up while doing them. It provides a positive interruption of our daily routine.

First, these are some of the things you should watch out for while doing your exercises:

- The right posture. Do not tense up while standing but remain loose, with your knees slightly bent. Stand with your legs slightly apart. Keep your legs shoulder-width apart.
- Breathe correctly. Try to breathe calmly and steadily. This helps you to relax.
- Proper concentration. Don't let yourself be distracted by anything.
- Proper preparation. Don't jump out of your chair and start with the exercises. Take some time to collect yourself.
- Unwind properly. Close your eyes during exercise. You might have difficulty at the beginning but closing your eyes increases the tension relief.

Exercise 1: Relieving Tension in Your Feet

Try to make a fist with your toes. Keep the tension for a few seconds, then quickly release them. Relax for a few minutes and then repeat the exercise.

Exercise 2: Relieving Tension in Your Legs

Stretch your knees completely so your legs are straight. Tighten the muscles in your upper and lower legs as much as you can. Keep the tension for a short period and then abruptly release. Relax a bit and then repeat the exercise.

Exercise 3: Relieving Tension in the Buttocks

Tighten your buttocks with all your strength for a few seconds. Then relieve the tension abruptly. After a short break repeat the exercise.

Exercise 4: Relieving Stomach Tension

Push your stomach out as far as you can. Breathe in while you're doing this. Hold this position for a few seconds. Then relieve the tension abruptly, breathing out at the same time. Take a short break and then repeat the exercise.

Exercise 5: Relieving Back Tension

Arch your back like a cat. Relax after a few seconds in this position. Wait a bit and then repeat the exercise.

Exercise 6: Relieving Chest Tension

Breathe in deeply and hold the air in for a few seconds, then abruptly breathe out. Take a short break and then repeat.

Exercise 7: Relieving Shoulder Tension

With all your strength, push your shoulders back as far as you can. Keep them there for a few seconds and abruptly let go. After a short break repeat the exercise, pushing your shoulders up or to the front.

Exercise 8: Relieving Facial Tension

Tighten the muscles of your face into a grimace. Keep the tension up for a few seconds and then abruptly let go again.

> *You can do this "fitness training" while on the phone.*

I recently discovered an alternative to office exercises in an American magazine. These exercises were designed for the time you waste while "on hold" on the phone. We spend an average of 15 minutes a day on hold. So here are some exercises you can do while stuck in a "holding pattern."

Exercise 1: The Tennis Ball Trick

Hold a tennis ball and squeeze it as hard as you can. After two seconds, release it. You should do this 30 times with each hand.

Exercise 2: The Book Trick

Take a book in your right hand and lift it over your head until your arm is fully stretched. Make sure your palm is facing forward. Then bend your arm and bring the book behind your head. Do this 20 times with each arm.

Exercise 3: The Desk Trick

Stand up and hook your right foot around your left ankle. Holding on to your desk, flex your left foot slowly up and down, so that you are up on your toes, then down again. Repeat this 30 times and then do the same thing with your other leg.

Exercise 4: The Paper Trick

This is a seated exercise. Take a stack of papers and hold them in one hand, palm up. Your arm should rest on your upper thigh so that your wrist touches your knee cap. Grasping the stack of paper, flex your wrist to move it up and down. Repeat this 10 or 15 times and then do it with your other hand.

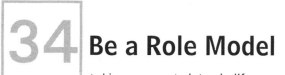

34 Be a Role Model

Taking up sports later in life can extend
your life for many years and help you become
a hero to the younger generation.

I t's never too late to drop that sedentary lifestyle and start exercising.

> *More than half the children in the United States take part in no sport at all.*

Many studies have concluded that:

- Fitness training should begin at an early age.
- Exercise can be very beneficial even in old age.
- Exercise can have positive effects even when begun at 70.

Why should we interest our children in sports? There are many reasons. The most important being: sport is fun for most kids. They make new friends, they quickly learn the rules of competition, experience the feeling of success, and the lesson of losing every now and then. Children who participate in sport are happier, more balanced, and meet with more success later in life.

Sporty children, however, achieve something even more important: they're healthy. Naturally, heart ailments and even heart attacks are comparatively rare in children, but an increasing number of studies conclude that heart and circulatory ailments can take root at an early age. The American Heart Association has released alarming facts concerning the state of health of our youngsters (American in this case, but the rest of the Western world is unfortunately not far behind):

- More than half the children going to American schools do no sport at all.
- Sports-shy children have a higher cholesterol level, higher blood pressure and a lower level of the heart-protective cholesterol HDL in their blood.
- The number of obese children between the ages of 6 and 12 has increased 54% since 1960. In the age group between 12 and 17, it has increased by 39%.
- 14.2 million girls and 12.8 million boys under the age of 19 in the U.S. have a cholesterol level of 170 mg/dl and above. In hardly any other country in the world do children have worse blood fat levels.
- 2.1 million children smoke. Nine million children live in homes where at least one person smokes.
- Children spend an average of 17 hours a week in front of the television. This figure does not take computers, video games, or the Internet into account.

Many young people lead a life that is filled with classic high-risk factors for heart and circulatory illnesses: smoking, bad cholesterol levels, not enough exercise, and obesity.

I have personally experienced how important parents are as role models for their children. I learned from my mother how to relax with music, and from my father how to have a healthy diet. There is only one way to make our children healthier: be a role model yourself. You can't buy exercise at the supermarket; you have to grow up with it.

Sport Rejuvenates

If you get your children or grandchildren to participate in sport it will have a positive effect on you as well. An increasing number of studies has confirmed the importance of exercise later in life. And it doesn't make a bit of difference if you exercised in your youth or not. Even if you start exercising late in life you can extend your life expectancy by many years.

> *Try above all to slow down the loss of muscle fiber.*

A person starts losing muscle fiber in the body from about the age of 30, on average about 6% every 10 years. The most rapid decrease takes place in the muscle fibers responsible for speed. This is the reason why there are many long-distance runners in their forties but no sprinters over the age of 35.

The decrease in the slower muscle fibers is a longer process and therefore can more easily be reversed. Endurance training is one of the best methods. This includes sports like swimming, hiking, jogging, and cross-country skiing.

An increasing number of older people are spending more and more time in front of the television. They walk less, go on fewer excursions, and travel less compared to the early 1980s. This was revealed in a study done by the B.A.T. Recreational Research Institute (Freizeits-forschungsinsitut) in Hamburg, Germany. One in three pensioners spends the afternoons watching television. In 1983 only 12% watched the television during these hours of the day.

Wildor Hollman, a sports physician from Cologne, proved how effective endurance training can be for older people. Through specific exercise programs, 60- to 70-year-olds – even if they have not been physically active for decades – can reach the performance levels of 40-year-olds. Even the life expectancy of 70- to 80-year-olds can be extended with these exercise programs. Parallel to this, their oxygen intake is increased, thereby improving mental capacity and reinvigorating the immune system.

> *Every third pensioner spends the afternoon in front of the television.*

Wildor Hollman concludes: "Were there a medicine that could provide all these positive effects it would be the discovery of the century. Sadly, however, its widespread use is dependent on the physical law of inertia."

35 Donate Blood

Giving blood not only helps to save
a stranger's life, but can protect your own.

In the United States over 8 million people a year donate blood. In Britain it's 1.8 million. Most people donate blood because they want to help others. New research shows you just might be helping yourself the most.

Giving blood is a tradition hundreds of years old. Most likely it was doctors in India who first used "blood-letting" as a method of cleansing the body. However, even Hippocrates termed blood-letting one of the most important healing methods for acute illnesses. Blood was taken, above all, when diseases of the lung, the brain, and the heart were diagnosed. In early times it was a dangerous procedure, the patient very often paying with his life.

In the twentieth century blood-letting was virtually forgotten. For a long time its purpose was disputed. In the light of the current trend for rediscovering ancient natural healing methods, an increasing number of doctors have re-established the value of blood-letting. For the first time there are also conclusive research studies to back up the value of giving blood.

A study at the University of Kansas was able to come up with evidence that giving blood regularly can lower the heart attack risk – particularly in men. A research team checked the condition of the heart and arteries of 655 men and women over 40 years of age who regularly gave blood. These results were compared to blood tests of 3,200 people who never gave blood. The result was that the regular male blood donors suffered 30% less from clogged arteries or a heart attack in comparison to non-donors. Among women and smokers the positive effects of giving blood could not be conclusively verified.

> *Male blood donors in the U.S. had a 30% reduced risk of heart attack.*

The American Journal of Epidemiology recently reported on a study in Finland. Researchers at the University of Kuopio found evidence that giving blood can reduce the heart attack risk in males. For the study, the medical profiles of 3,000 males were compared. In the blood-donor group, only 0.7% had suffered a heart attack. The rate among non-donors was 12%.

Why Giving Blood Is a Good Thing

There is still too little research concerning the true effects of giving blood. The Finnish researchers believe the heart attack risk increases with the amount of iron in the blood. People who regularly give blood reduce their blood iron (ferrite) levels without any signs of deficiency. Ferriten is a protein that binds iron in the blood. A ferrite level of 200 or above doubles the risk of a heart attack. A lower level, on the other hand, has a positive effect on cholesterol and on the metabolism, thereby protecting the body from deposits of artery-hardening substances. This reduces the risk of heart attacks and strokes.

> *Giving blood lowers the ferrite level in your blood. A low ferrite level is good for the heart.*

American researchers are searching for further positive effects of donating blood. More than 1.5 million Americans suffer from haemochromatosis, a genetic iron-retaining condition in which organs retain too much iron. This can result in impotence, diabetes, sterility, severe liver damage, and even death. Men under 50 are five times more likely to suffer from this illness than women. If the disease is detected early, blood donations can help before the damage to the body is too great.

I think it is too early to tell conclusively if giving blood actually protects the heart. Perhaps people who donate blood live healthier lives anyway, and therefore have a lower heart attack risk. But what does that change? Do we really need to know the reason why we're healthy? The concept of giving blood can perhaps be compared to a healthy diet. Not everyone who switches to healthy food will be able to reduce cholesterol levels radically. But a healthy diet has an array of other benefits in the battle against heart disease: lower weight, lower blood pressure, and overall well-being. By regularly giving blood we will not necessarily protect the heart directly. But it is a first, active step in the battle against a heart attack – a step in the direction of better health.

36 Enjoy Sex

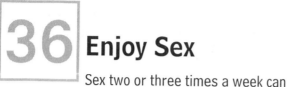

Sex two or three times a week can lengthen your life. More often, though, is bad for your immune system.

Over the course of the past 30 years, thousands of newspaper reports about me have been published. Many have been serious, some not so, and a few unintentionally funny. Recently in a respected German newspaper I read the following description of me: "He is a doctor of the old school. They were men who stood as ardently in surgery as they drove fast cars and indulged in tumultuous love affairs." What absolute rubbish! I never had a fast car and did not have sex until I was 25 – older than most of my contemporaries – and that was with my first wife. I was part of a generation that still placed a certain value on waiting until marriage before having sex.

> *The media like to portray me as a Don Juan. In fact, I had my first sexual experience at 25.*

As a student I had no fear of sex. The only fear I had was failing my exams. Every day I studied was a financial burden for the poor missionary family Barnard.

Now let me set the record straight. Sex is and always was a very important part of life for me. Sex always meant many things to me: love of my partner, pleasure, relaxation, and activity – much better than all that mindless jogging. It also protects against a heart attack, as a recent study concerning the connection between sex and death rates has revealed. In a cooperative research study by the universities of Bristol and Belfast, Professors Davey Smith, Stephen Frankel, and John Yarnell examined 918 Welshmen between the ages of 45 and 59 in the small town of Caerphilly and five neighboring communities. The results of this 10-year study provided the basis for an interesting theory:

- Sexually active men live longer.

The researchers divided the men into two groups. The representatives of the "low sex" group maintained that they had only about one orgasm per month. The "high sex" group assured the researchers that they had sex at least twice a week. Even taking into account other risk factors such as smoking, high blood pressure, stress, and cholesterol, the results were clear. In the "high sex" group of men the death rate risk factor was less than half that of the first group. It's no wonder that the university colleagues demanded in a British scientific journal that a national campaign be initiated. The reason: the health advantages of sex are too little known and must be made public.

Sex Helps Prevent Influenza

Americans should heed this advice too, because a study undertaken in the U.S. under completely different circumstances came to virtually the same results. Carl Charnetski and Frank Brennan of Wilkes University in Pennsylvania examined students between the ages of 16 and 23 years of age. The result: students who had sex twice a week had a much better developed immune system. Researchers found that they had a higher concentration (up to 30% higher) of immunoglobulin A (IgA) in their saliva. This is an antibody found in the blood, in the mucous membrane, and in numerous body fluids, and is part of the body's defence against many infections and poisonous substances. Its "speciality": fighting off influenza and colds.

> *If you have more sex, you will strengthen your body's defence system.*

Moderate sexual activity leads to a stimulation of the IgA production. Therefore the immunologist Clifford Lowell of the University of San Francisco concludes: "It's easily possible that the immune system is stimulated through moderate body contact, because during each such contact germ cells are transferred." What's puzzling is another test result: in everyone who has sex more than three times a week, the IgA concentration rapidly diminishes. Perhaps it is as I have long thought it to be: sex is not just an exchange of body fluids; it is also an emotional experience. It's possible that in those who have sex more than three times a week the emotional component is lacking – the perfect playing ground for stress and fear. Even though science is still somewhat in the dark concerning this, one thing has been empirically proven: stress and fear not only foster the possibility of a heart attack but they also lead to a general reduction of IgA, thereby causing a weakening of the body's defence system.

> *Sex is not some new type of competitive sport. It is the most beautiful experience in the world.*

Sex, regular sex, is the most beautiful, healthiest, and most pleasurable way to keep the circulation in gear, keeping the heart healthy. There should be no "rules" for how often you should have sex. Just try to observe two essentials:

1 You should always have sex when there is a natural need for it.
2 You should never have sex when it feels like a chore or a performance. Our achievement-oriented society has spoiled enough of life's pleasures; don't let sex be one of them.

I have also developed a few additional principles. It's possible I might have created them from my subconscious and my experience:

• Never have sex outside the bedroom.
• Never have sex in strange beds.
• Never pay for sex.

I am more of a romantic lover. Perhaps many will laugh at this description, but I believe it and refer exclusively to personal experience: I never just "needed" sex enough to pay for it. I can even recall a very unpleasant experience concerning this subject back in 1963. I had just arrived in the city of light, Paris, from a very depressing Moscow during Cold War times. As I was walking along the Champs-Elysées I encountered an attractive woman who gave me a friendly smile. We got conversing and suddenly, out of the blue, she asked me to come to a hotel with her. I agreed and we went to a small, clean, and discreet hotel. It was so discreet that I almost didn't notice the "spy" who was observing us in the foyer through a keyhole in a wooden door.

Upon entering the room the attractive young woman immediately began undressing. I said: "No, no, that's not the way I want to do it. I would like to talk with you some more first." She replied: "Talk? Well, OK, but that will cost you more." I quickly left the room. Even the "spy" was surprised. He opened his door and yelled after me: "That was the quickest session we ever had in this house!"

Sex in Later Life Is Important

I have had a lot of sex in my life, and the older I got the more important it became for me. However, I believe that sex should always be in the context of a love affair – however short-lived or minor. This may sound a bit strange coming from a man who has always been described by the media as a kind of "womanizer." But I ask you to believe me when I say that a married man should try to be faithful. That is my firm conviction. I realize today that my marriages never ended because of unfaithfulness but only because I neglected my partner at the time. It's important for couples to keep sexuality "alive," never stop being creative, and never stop making sex interesting. Many couples no longer enjoy sex because they have stopped making it interesting or trying to think of something new to stimulate themselves. By the way, just this lack of creativity can be responsible for sexual problems. There is a saying which quite accurately describes this: "Use it or lose it."

Sex, it is frequently said, is taking over our society. I don't think this is true; it is certainly exaggerated. There is still little sex on television when compared to the frequent scenes of brutality. I would prefer our children to see more sex than violence on TV.

The dangers for our children today lie elsewhere. If I could give the youth of today some recommendations concerning this, they would be as follows:

- Be careful when you have sex with a new partner. Use a condom, even though sex might be less fun with it.
- If you decide on a long-term relationship then both of you should take an AIDS test in order to enjoy the relationship without fear.
- One can no longer say as a parent today that youngsters should wait until they're married to have sex. One can only tell them that they should at least like the person they're having sex with, and that that person should like – and respect – them.

I think that a healthy sexuality not only helps strengthen the heart and protect against a heart attack but is good for one's soul. It's no accident that in the United States, where the feelings surrounding sex contrast most (anything from complete sexual freedom to the most extreme form of prudery can be found), a recent study caused an uproar. According to findings published by the University of Chicago, one in three Americans has major problems with his or her sexuality. Professor Edward Laumann came to the conclusion – after examining 1,749 women and 1,410 men between the ages of 18 and 59 – that "sexual disturbances are wide-spread."

> *Every third American has serious problems with his or her sexuality.*

A particularly interesting aspect of the study was the varying curves of "pleasure." The findings showed that women were finding more joy in sex as they got older, while for men of the same age the pleasure was rapidly declining. The proportion of sexually unhappy men in these age groups rose by an astounding 300%.

Barnard Tips for a Healthy Heart

What Good Sex Can Do for You

1 **Sex is love.**

   There should always be a little love affair involved with sex.

2 **Sex is rejuvenation.**

   Strictly speaking, it's a sporting activity. And activity always keeps you young.

3 **Sex is health.**

   Take the studies seriously: sexually active people live longer.

4 **Sex is a generator of ideas.**

   Remaining sexually creative will also help you to bring more creativity into the rest of your life.

5 **Sex is a test.**

   I may be old-fashioned: I think partners should try to remain faithful.

6 **Sex is training.**

   Good sex is the best heart and cardiovascular activity!

7 **Sex is a good teacher.**

   Try not to behave worse in bed than in the rest of your life.

8 **Sex is not a financial matter.**

   Of course money buys you anything today, but does this make every investment a good one?

9 **Sex is not a competitive sport.**

   If you absolutely have to do it in the elevator or on a plane, OK, but that's really about bragging later on, isn't it?

10 **Sex is exercise.**

   If you don't train regularly you soon won't have any strength left in your muscles.

37 | Keep Walking

Walking is the best way to better health.
For every 800 yards you walk, your chances
of a heart attack diminish by 15% .

I am acquainted with a well-known European publisher who has placed his telephone at the very corner of his rather sparsely furnished office. Between his desk and the telephone there is a space of at least four yards. When I expressed surprise at this, the man – who today is in his seventies – told me, with a twinkle in his eye, the reason for this: "Naturally I could put the telephone on my desk, but like this I am forced to get up and walk a few yards every time it rings."

This gentleman integrated physical activity into his daily routine, and I could only congratulate him for taking this step. This is a decision that anyone can vary according to his or her taste and make it a "subconscious" form of exercise. It doesn't always have to be that controversial activity, jogging (very frequently done improperly) that keeps you in shape. Simple everyday movements can do the same for you. Climbing stairs, playing with the children, taking the dog for a walk, or cutting the grass – everything that keeps you moving can serve as part of your personal fitness program.

> *If you walk two miles every day, you will lower your risk of getting a heart attack by 50%.*

A research study published by the University of Washington came to sensational conclusions: 2,678 men between the ages of 71 and 93 were asked about their daily walking habits. Those who walked an average of two miles a day lowered their risk of a heart attack by more than 50% compared to those who only walked about 400 yards a day. Another astounding fact revealed by this study was that for every 800 yards walked per day, the heart attack risk sank by 15%.

The scientific journal which published these findings also published a commentary by two physicians from the University of Texas at Austin, Peter Snell and Jahre Mitchell. They said it was extremely encouraging that one could reduce the risk of a heart attack with so little effort and in such a short time.

Did you know that one of America's fastest-growing new sports was invented in Germany? While still at school, American Gary Yanker visited the Black Forest and joined a hiking club there. Twenty years later he became the guru of a new fitness trend in the U.S.: (fast) walking. "I got the idea in Germany," Yanker says today. "That is where I discovered my love of hiking. I went on many tours with the German Boy Scouts, including one to Lake Constance."

> *America's latest fitness trend was invented in Germany: fast walking.*

Walking is a classic form of sport that you can do every day. You don't need to buy any fitness apparatus, you don't even need special clothes for it. You can walk to your place of work (45–60 steps per minute), go walking with your family (45 steps per minute) or you can look upon it as an alternative to jogging. When "speed walking" you take 100–160 steps per minute. The effect is always the same. You burn fat, strengthen your muscles (without straining any joints) and help your cardiovascular system.

Because it is so simple and places fewer demands on the body than jogging, walking is finding more and more adherents. Often the reasons given for not doing exercise are quite simple ones. We don't want to spend money on fitness studio membership or we don't have the time to go to the swimming pool. So we do nothing. A better idea: you build sport into your daily life and make a ritual

of it. Our whole life is full of such habits. Just think: the way you prepare for work every morning, how you arrange your day, how you
get ready to go to bed in the evening. It's all habit and ritual.

> *Make sport an everyday ritual – like eating or brushing your teeth.*

You can do this with activity too. Draw up a schedule for yourself.
Example: when you come home from work, play with the children
for 10 minutes. Or: from now on get up 15 minutes earlier and go
(on foot!) to buy a newspaper.

What sort of activity you take up is not nearly as important as
the fact that you're being active. The Centers for Disease Control in
Washington reported that "laziness" constitutes the same risk
factors for a heart attack as high blood pressure, "bad" cholesterol,
or cigarettes.

Now one would think that a person made aware of such pro-
found studies would not be stupid enough to ignore them. But
knowing is apparently not enough – we need further motivation,
in black and white.

At least this was the conclusion of a study undertaken in Auck-
land, New Zealand. They found that verbal recommendations
from doctors to their patients concerning exercise were less likely
to be heeded than a written prescription.

> *Let your doctor prescribe sport for you. That will really get you
> moving.*

In total the researchers examined the behaviour of 456 New
Zealand patients who, due to lack of exercise, were in a high-risk
group for heart disease. Over 220 received written prescriptions
on what to do, the other half received only verbal recommendations. The result was that of those who were "prescribed" exercise, 80 began immediately to start their fitness training; in the
"verbal" group, only 48 did the same.

What your "prescription" on how you can minimize your heart
attack risk should look like:

- Add physical activity to your routine at work. Make telephone calls while you're standing. Don't take the elevator – walk.
- Make it a ritual to take a regular daily walk of at least 800 yards and you will reduce your heart attack risk by 15%.
- Avoid psychological barriers to physical activity. Don't think you have to go to a pool or a fitness center in order to get active.

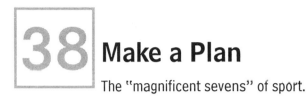

38 Make a Plan

The "magnificent sevens" of sport.

Activity once a day can reduce the chance of having a heart attack by an incredible 45%. It's as simple as that. To get there you don't have to jog 50 times around the block, take your dog for a fast walk up a mountain, or work out for three hours in a fitness studio.

Relatively moderate physical activity can almost halve the risk of cardiovascular disease. Such activity could be:

1 washing your car for 45 minutes
2 cleaning your windows for 45 minutes
3 30 minutes of gardening
4 15 minutes of shovelling snow
5 skipping for 15 minutes
6 mowing your lawn for 30 minutes
7 dancing for 30 minutes.

OK, not everybody can be John Travolta. And perhaps you don't have a garden – or a car. Then you might have to make it a traditional sport. That's OK too. First of all you should sit down for a few minutes and think about what sort of activity would be best for you. How much time do you have at your disposal? What do you like doing? In what physical condition are you? Last, not least, are you a social animal or do you take more pleasure from performing solo?

> *Washing your car or shovelling snow can halve your risk of a heart attack.*

Before you begin with a plan of activity, you should have found answers to the following seven questions:

1   How fit are you?
2   How old are you?
3   What do you expect to gain from sport?
4   Do you want to go it alone or join a group?
5   Do you prefer to do your work-out in the open air or behind closed doors?
6   How much money are you prepared to spend on this?
7   How does sport fit into your daily life?

If you have not done any sport for a long time and are over 40 years old, you should first seek the approval of your doctor before you commence your exercise program. You may find that you have a latent heart problem which, while not affecting you in your normal daily life, may become dangerous when you begin to do sport. Get yourself checked, but in any case begin your activity gently, regardless of whether this is a true beginning or just a new start after a long break. Don't open your innings with a marathon – walking a few hundred yards at first is more likely to be good for you. Or swimming just a few lengths. Increase whatever activity you have decided to take up gradually.

> *Don't just go from 0 to 60. Build up your body gradually.*

Good training is not a rigorous science but a matter of adhering to some simple rules. Warm up well, note your pulse at regular intervals, learn to relax fully between activities. If you make these three aspects a routine part of your activity, you won't overtax your body and you will get more pleasure out of all that you do.

Before putting on your jogging shoes you should have found your own answers to the following questions:

1 What is the best way for you to become fit?
2 How hard should you train?
3 How long should you train?
4 How long should you warm up (and cool off)?
5 How often should you train?
6 What happens when you miss a few training sessions?
7 Is there a limit to training?

A good fitness program is a long-term arrangement. Don't expect of the sport what it cannot deliver. A month's training will not enable you to take on the triathlon. You must conceive a fitness plan for yourself which provides for a steady increase in activity. You should train regularly, otherwise you will soon be back to square one. Begin with 15-minute sessions three times a week and increase to 30 minutes when you feel right for it. You fix your limit. If after some weeks you feel ready for an hour's training (sport or exercise), then you should go for it.

> *Regular training can save you 13 million heartbeats a year.*

Training is not: drive somewhere – get out of the car – jog – get into the car – drive home. Five minutes' warm-up and five minutes' cooling off time are essential. Your body isn't a motor which is simply started and stopped.

Don't think that exercise means only your arms and legs. Success is determined by the extent to which you consider your heart. The American Heart Association has determined that the heart of a fit person beating 50 times a minute pumps as much blood into the body as the heart of an unfit person does with 70 beats a minute. In this way active, fit people can save their heart 13 million beats a year.

YOUR FINAL PULSE RATE
How Sport Can Put the Right Demands on Your Heart

To train your heart optimally, your pulse while doing sport (known as your final pulse rate, the one to aim for) should reach 50 to 75% of your maximum heart rate. The formula for calculating your maximum heart rate: 220 minus your age.

Age	30
Maximum heart rate	190 beats a minute
Final pulse rate	95—142 beats a minute
Age	35
Maximum heart rate	185 beats a minute
Final pulse rate	93—138 beats a minute

> *You are 60? Then your heart rate should not be faster than 120 beats a minute during sport.*

Age	40
Maximum heart rate	180 beats a minute
Final pulse rate	90—135 beats a minute
Age	45
Maximum heart rate	175 beats a minute
Final pulse rate	88—131 beats a minute
Age	50
Maximum heart rate	170 beats a minute
Final pulse rate	85—127 beats a minute
Age	55
Maximum heart rate	165 beats a minute
Final pulse rate	83—123 beats a minute
Age	60
Maximum heart rate	160 beats a minute
Final pulse rate	80—120 beats a minute

Age	65
Maximum heart rate	155 beats a minute
Final pulse rate	78—116 beats a minute

Age	70
Maximum heart rate	150 beats a minute
Final pulse rate	75—112 beats a minute

You should always train in such a way that you place a maximum demand of 75% on your heart. That means, as the above table indicates, that there is a maximum heart rate for every age. The average heart cannot beat faster than this. You can easily calculate your maximum heart rate: 220 minus your age. So if you are 60, your maximum is 160 beats a minute.

> *Optimal training raises your heart rate to 75% of its maximum capacity. More than that can cause damage, less is ineffectual.*

If you want to train your heart optimally, your pulse should never beat faster than between 50 and 75% of your maximum heart rate. In the case of a 60-year-old this would be between 80 and 120 beats a minute. This is known as the final pulse rate: the one to aim for. Too much can do damage, too little is almost useless. If you place too little demand on your heart (less than 50% of maximum), your training will not be of much use.

It is important to know how to train your body optimally. Wrong sport can be worse for you than no sport at all. When you carry out a training plan you should have thought of an answer to the following questions:

1 Am I overexerting myself?
2 Am I keeping a proper eye on my body?
3 Am I reaching the right heart rate?
4 Am I sufficiently prepared for what I am doing?
5 Do I eat in accordance with my activity?
6 Does what I do suit my type of body?
7 Am I making the correct movements?

OK, now you are hard at work. But what do you get from that? A good mood, self-confidence, perhaps new friends. But wasn't there something else? Of course: weight loss. Doing sport burns up fat. If you don't follow up your training with potato chips and beer, then your new desire for movement will have a positive effect on your waistline and your weight will go down. The following table will show you how many calories a man weighing 165 pounds can burn up in an hour. If you weigh more, you burn up more.

Sport	Calories/Hour
Walking (4 miles)	440
Walking (2 miles)	240
Skipping (rope)	750
Running (7 miles)	920
Long-distance skiing	700
Swimming (1 mile)	275
Swimming (2 miles)	500
Tennis (singles)	400
Cycling (12 miles)	410

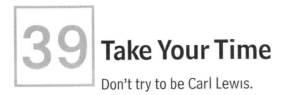

39 | Take Your Time

Don't try to be Carl Lewis.

Movement is good for the heart, that is clear. But I must warn you: Anyone who makes their exercise program part of contemporary society's almost bitter obsession with competition is not going to reduce their heart attack risk one bit. On the contrary, it will increase. A quick dash to the tennis court and then a rush back to the office is dangerous and cannot be considered good for one's health. Heart attacks are rare on the tennis court or in the swimming pool, but they keep on occurring directly after sport.

If you want to become active, you must make enough time for it. If you constantly get to the golf course, the ski run, or the squash court at the last minute or even later, then you should honestly admit to yourself that you don't have the time for these sports. Try doing something else such as walking, swimming, or long-distance skiing. Thirty minutes three times per week are enough. Use the time you gain by changing your routine to prepare yourself properly for these 30 minutes. That will enhance your health.

When jogging was the rage there were many – this I know from personal experience – who hated it but did it none the less. After all, it was in fashion. Running has a few "built-in" risk factors, however, for trained and untrained participants alike. But hardly anyone is aware of these.

Risk 1   Very few people really have the body of a runner, a body which makes jogging the ideal sport for them. A jogger places four times his normal body weight on his joints. Because of the way we are built, only 10% of us will have absolutely no problems with jogging.

Risk 2   Many people treat the dangers associated with great bodily effort very lightly. Consider the following: studies on marathon runners have shown that during a run the immune system can briefly be reduced to dangerously low defence levels.

Sport deserves the proper amount of time, otherwise it will not only be of no benefit but can actually become harmful.

- Take the time to prepare yourself emotionally for sport. What use is it if you train for all you are worth while your mind is still on your work?
- Take the time to warm up properly. Not doing so is the worst of all sport sins: onto the court, racquet in hand, ready to slam the first ball into your opponent's left corner. Not even your car would survive such treatment.
- Take the time to do sport. Don't keep looking at your watch. If you can find no time for a sport, you shouldn't try to do it.
- Take the time to recover from sport. Your blood pressure is still very high, your heart is pumping for dear life – but you pretend it was nothing, a piece of cake. Give your body time to regain its normal working temperature.

Sport and stress have a close working relationship. I would like to demonstrate this to you with an example. In the 1980s the world-renowned conductor, Herbert von Karajan, made himself available to a scientific research study in Salzburg concerning itself with the combination of emotional stress and physical activity. His heart rate during various activities, such as flying a plane (his private jet), driving a car, and conducting, was among the many reactions that were measured.

> *Herbert von Karajan conducted with a heart rate of up to 200 – until he was 80.*

The results were astounding: during a Beethoven piece the maestro reached a rate of up to 200 heartbeats a minute, a rate that would usually send all medical alarm bells ringing. But Herbert von Karajan managed to conduct excellently under these circumstances, and he stayed healthy until he died – at 80. Why? Because stress and activity go together perfectly. Stress causes our body to produce certain hormones. Of particular importance for the heart are the catecholamines, which in turn are decomposed in the mitochondria. People doing sport have more mitochondria and can therefore overcome stress more rapidly.

While conducting, Herbert von Karajan unconsciously did the very thing that has become part of the standard repertoire of every school of management: stress is neutralized through sport. Karajan's conducting, although very stressful, was also a sporting activity.

40 Be Creative

Approach sport as you approach sex:
keep on thinking of something new to do.

Towards the end of the 1980s the American Heart Association created a sensation. Its experts published a research study that was very critical of American youth – and particularly of their parents. The study concluded that 50% of the children and young adults tested did not participate in any form of physical activity that could be seen as long-term protection against heart disease. Another study of grade school children provided even worse results: 36% of schools did not even offer physical education classes as part of the curriculum!

These findings were particularly disturbing considering the American Heart Association's estimation that at the time the number of deaths at all ages attributed to the lack of physical fitness was 250,000 per year.

This was after American health authorities had propagated for years that activity programs should "keep it simple." Even a minimal amount of physical activity could reduce the heart attack risk by 25%. Neither parachuting nor mountain biking, but simple things like walking up steps, working around the house, dancing, and even doing housework were among the recommendations.

Anyone doing some physical activity every day – regardless of which age you start – will be rewarded by 10 improvements in the body, which also will improve your sense of well-being and your mood. It's hard to believe what can be achieved by regularly doing things like climbing steps, gardening, or doing household chores:

1 Circulation is improved and the heart attack risk is reduced.
2 Your weight can more easily be kept under control.
3 Your cholesterol level can be improved.
4 Activity: the perfect protection against osteoporosis.
5 It's an ideal way to combat depression and bouts of fear or anxiety.
6 Your optimism and enthusiasm increase.
7 Activity combats high blood pressure.
8 It provides you with more energy and is the ideal form of stress management.
9 It increases self-confidence.
10 It helps you to sleep better.

The first people to achieve this were managers of U.S. companies. The bodily fitness of upper management has come to be looked upon as part of an enterprise's capital assets. Paging through a few business magazines will show that the traditional overweight manager no longer exists. Today top executives strive to look like Michael Eisner, top man in the Disney corporation. Slimness suggests dynamism. Fitness reflects a self-assured presence, creativity, competence in problem-solving, and resilience against stress. These are characteristics required increasingly of top executives in business, industry, media, and politics.

> *Today's manager is slim, demonstrating drive and forcefulness.*

Sport Makes You Creative

Findings from a study done at the University of Middlesex provided evidence that physical activity also stimulates creativity. Two groups of the same size were given a creative task to perform – but beforehand one group had had a half-hour of exercise, the other had sat and watched videos. The task was to build a tower out of cardboard boxes and empty tins. The group who had exercised won by a mile. Their fantasy tower could not be matched by their "couch potato" competitors.

Even the argument that sport would overtax the "time budget" of a top executive has no bearing here. A top management executive who participates in a sport three times a week for 30 to 60 minutes is much more effective and quicker in his or her decision-making due to increased performance capabilities. The two to three hours a week "spent" on activity are quickly made up for by a more efficient and faster work pace. He or she probably even gains time.

> *In sport as in sex – you're either creative or bored.*

If it isn't lack of time which keeps us from doing sport, what is it? Perhaps the fact that many people find sport too boring. To run mile after mile in a gym or in the open, or to swim one length after another may not at first seem like a form of entertainment which one could put up with for a long time. But there is a simple trick for eliminating boredom in sport: create diversions for yourself. Don't always run the same route, don't only do *one* sport but rather mix a few disciplines. Create a few positive rituals which you associate with movement – you might, for instance, use your sport to make or meet friends. You will see: sport is a bit like sex, it can become boring if you can't think of new things to do.

A person wanting to be healthy later in life must not only train their muscles but also their coordination abilities. One should consistently learn new movements and then use these in competitive situations. As strange as it sounds, this can be of life-saving importance in old age. Because a well-trained, coordinated body is a good way to prevent falls. As we all know, the notorious broken hip has dramatically changed the life of many an older person. If you remain agile, you are far less likely to fall.

> *Don't laugh about golf. It is possibly the best preventive sport against heart attacks.*

The Viennese sports physician Professor Bachl has taken a critical look at sports for better fitness and as a heart protector. In his opinion some sports – certain types of games – must be considered with caution. There is nothing against tennis if it is played in moderation. "It is important to find a healthy balance in the game and not add to stress. So it is good just to practice for a bit, or take some lessons every now and then, rather than always playing a game and subjecting oneself to the stress of competition."

For middle-aged people he recommends golf, a sport which is now taken seriously by many: "It's an excellent form of prevention even if it is laughed at and downplayed as a real sport. One walks at a rather brisk pace for a good 4 miles in healthy surroundings when playing 18 holes while towing a bag of clubs. This is a very effective exercise program."

Instead of an injury-prone sport, Bachl recommends table tennis. Why? It can be played virtually without risk and is a good way to improve muscle coordination. Swimming is an excellent form of exercise for healthy people. Twenty minutes of serious swimming can be better than or at least as good as running, and puts less pressure on your joints.

Your attitude is important for all sports: think positive. Sport isn't a bitter pill which you have to take whether you like it or not. Look on sport as neither more nor less than the only way in which you can be younger at heart than your sedentary contemporaries.

Attitude

41 Show Your Feelings

A good grip on your emotional
life makes you better able to
deal with physical problems.

There are a variety of strong connections between the psyche and heart attack risk. Countless studies undertaken at university clinics throughout the world have provided me with evidence of this. Naturally there has also been relevant research in Vienna, the "world capital of psychoanalysis." The renowned psychiatrist and university professor Stefan Rudas is in no doubt that a variety of psychological characteristics in a person can lead to either a higher or lower risk of cardiac arrest. A person with a frequent tendency to anxiety, to depression, or to hectic activity runs a greater risk of developing heart problems than a person with a tolerant, cheerful disposition.

> *I promise you: look after your soul and you will reduce your chances of a heart attack.*

The psyche controls our behavior and therefore the irresponsible way in which we live. However, the theory that a heart attack is exclusively and, in the end, a final symptom of notorious behavioral disturbances is something I cannot accept without question. I don't believe that in a completely healthy, fit person psychological factors alone can lead to a heart attack. But I am sure that behavioral disturbances over a long period of time can cause organic illnesses.

I want to tell you a story about an acquaintance of mine which underscores the opinion that the psyche and the risk of falling ill can interlock.

This person, a renowned author, suffered between the ages of 20 and 30 from a rare but not medically unknown phenomenon: he had a pathological fear of dying from a heart attack.

Physically he was completely healthy, which his various check-ups proved. Once he was even taken to the intensive care unit of a hospital and, after a thorough examination, he was released within 48 hours. He was found to be organically completely healthy. Despite this he thought at least two dozen times a year that his last hour had come. It was quite unbelievable – the superficial symptoms that he felt during his panic attacks were similar to those experienced during a heart attack: chest pains, numbness in the left arm, and cold sweat over the whole body.

> *An author who suffered for 10 years from the fear that he would very soon die of a heart attack was cured in a strange and wonderful way.*

It was not possible later to determine exactly if these psychosomatic symptoms were subconsciously acquired through reading or actually occurred "naturally" through some psychologically-induced behavioral defect, because every time after he had survived a "close call" he voraciously read medical literature without, however, finding a satisfactory answer to his problems there.

Ten years' fear of death while physically in good shape – I can certainly empathize with him. The panic he must have felt throughout the 10 years even though his body was completely healthy must have been exceedingly exhausting. It would probably only have been a matter of time before these attacks actually caused real organic damage. But things turned out differently. The symptoms and his fear disappeared almost miraculously, thanks to one of the strangest "cures" I have ever heard of.

During the last years of his panic attacks the man started a family, moved into a house, and confronted his wife with his problems the moment they became acute. She was always fright-ened when the "attack" occurred, called a doctor or, for nights on end, guarded the bed of the man who appeared "close to dying."

> *"I think I am dying," he said. His wife simply turned over and slept on.*

The condition, which occurred mostly at night, would disappear again, usually after a night filled with worry and fear of death.

One night it happened again. The man once more felt the obvious heart attack symptoms, and with a weak hand shook his wife awake: "It's happening again, I think I'm dying, I only want to say goodbye …" His wife looked up momentarily, her face angry, and said only, "Do you know what time it is?" – it was 3.30 in the morning.

She then turned over on her side and went back to sleep. Her husband was flabbergasted at first, then angry. All kinds of feel-ings arose in him: irritation, consternation, and rage. He jumped out of bed, not knowing how to control his emotions. After about 10 minutes he had himself under control again. All of a sudden it occurred to him that during those 10 minutes he had felt all sorts of things but surely not the symptoms of a heart attack.

He drank a glass of water, went back to bed, and slept peace-fully until he was awakened by the morning sun.

After this experience he has never again come "close to death" from a "heart attack."

The man never found out what he had suffered from. Every doc-tor to whom he spoke about this only shrugged. Most of them thought of his experiences merely as an amusing anecdote. But there is really more to it than that. Samuel J. Mann, professor of clinical medicine at New York Hospital/Cornell Medical Center fre-quently found himself having to deal with people who imagined that they had dangerously high blood pressure or that they had cancer. This while there was nothing wrong with them at all. Pro-fessor Mann began to take a more active interest in these patients and he found that, in most cases, suppressed emotional problems were causing these imagined illnesses. In his book *Healing Hyper-tension: Uncovering the Secret Power of Your Hidden Emotion* he maintains that these unassimilated traumatic experiences could sometimes have occurred very long ago.

The psyche determines our daily life to a greater extent than we might suppose. This has many consequences including the risk of a heart attack.

- You have no control over your psyche.
  Everyone is different. Much of what we are is congenital. If you are psychologically inclined to take things more seriously, be in more of a hurry, and less able to give free rein to your feelings, then you run a greater risk of developing heart problems. Emotional problems can clearly raise the risk of cardiac arrest.
- You have full control over your psyche.
  You do not have to submit blindly to your fate. You can develop the power to reduce the risks to your heart. Approach your problems head on and don't make a secret of them. Be prepared to accept that your lifestyle (unhealthy eating habits, smoking, stress, too little physical activity) can influence your psyche. And change these bad habits as fast as you can.

Our jobs today have become very brutal. If I'm correctly interpreting current developments, there doesn't seem to be much hope on the horizon for things to get better. I consider ambition to be a useful quality, but you should not allow it to rule your life. I don't think that stress as such is bad, but it can play too big a role in our lives.

Developments in our time have created a type of person – the constant careerist – who is extremely at risk of having a heart attack.

These people get used to being under constant pressure at work and are not capable of shedding these symptoms of pressure in their private life. They always want to be someone else, someone "higher up" and do not accept the way they are. They cannot delegate and always have to do everything themselves.

> *Our world of work has created a new type of person: the constant careerist.*

In his studies, Professor Rudas was able to observe that the causes for this behavior can frequently be traced back to childhood. Often these sufferers were not loved or accepted for themselves as children but rather only for doing something "right" or for particularly good behavior. Anyone who as a child was always required to be diligent, well-behaved, and possibly even "better" than the rest, is, as an adult, in danger of having to go through life with this attitude of constantly having to fulfil some self-imposed duty for some selfless reason.

The Risk of the Constant Careerist

The organic consequences of this attitude are clearly evident. These people are constantly tense. In fact, in what should normally be regeneration phases, they produce even more stress hormones. Much more than the amount which, as we maintained in Part II, would be harmless and might even be useful. Why do they react this way? Because they are of the opinion that during the regeneration phase they are not being "diligent and well-behaved" but merely lazy – a bad conscience based on their experiences as a child. At such times of "laziness" they managed to impress or please their parents much less than usual.

The result is a vicious circle from which there seems to be no escape. Their dissatisfaction grows because they are never satisfied with themselves. Their organs "cramp up" – not only the stomach and intestines (which is bad enough) but also the heart and the circulatory and respiratory systems.

But in one's professional life the dangers don't lurk only on the rungs up the career ladder. The opposite experiences – being demoted or even fired – can be the final and triggering mechanism in a negative chain of events. The interaction of physical predisposition and psychic behavior patterns which makes conflict-solving more difficult, increases the risk of a heart attack considerably. Those who are unable to overcome psychological problems inevitably join the high-risk group.

How does one protect oneself against this? I believe there are three excellent preventive measures:

1 The courage to be imperfect.
   The risk of having a heart attack sinks dramatically if one has the courage to be imperfect. In other words: the courage to

accept the truth about ourselves – that we're as imperfect as everyone else. People at risk, in particular, must on occasion learn to accept even their second-best performance as sufficient. A person who is less hard on him- or herself is in less danger of "taking things to heart."

2 The courage to confess.
   Admit it when you have made a mistake. Nobody is perfect. A person who accepts his or her weaknesses actually gains in strength and self-confidence.

3 The courage to be honest.
   Don't avoid the issue. Face your problems and talk to others about them. That will reduce stress and give your heart the breathing space it needs.

> *If you can admit to weakness, you are really demonstrating strength.*

The American cardiologist Mark Ketterer of the Henry Ford Hospital in Detroit, Michigan, has shown how important it is that we sometimes give free rein to our feelings. Over a period of five years Ketterer examined 144 patients who were divided into two groups. The study concerned itself with getting people to discuss emotional stress. This included talking about suffering, sorrow and fear. The first group consisted of people who were able to talk freely about emotional problems. The second group tended to bottle up their emotional problems and to avoid talking about them.

> *If you suppress your emotional stress, you increase the risk of a heart attack.*

The amazing result was that five years later more than three dozen of the patients from the two groups had had heart attacks or other severe heart problems. But those who denied having emotional stress or did not speak about it had a much higher heart attack rate than those who did. Most of those who had heart problems were men. There is also a psychological reason for this. Our society expects men, as the "stronger" sex, to be better able to deal with emotional stress such as bereavement, fear, or sorrow on their own, without having to talk about it.

I think that our bodies sometimes function like steam engines. If you close the valve which releases the steam, the engine will at some time explode.

A person who cannot find a way to release pain, hurt, and disappointment forces the body to find a way sooner or later. It is usually a way that we do not like, because anyone trying to solve problems in this manner is on a dangerous path. Psychosomatic studies have shown that such a form of "coping with conflict" is the perfect example of an illness originating in the mind.

Many relationships, after a time, harbor unforeseen dangers caused by unresolved conflict. Yet in every long-term relationship there are things "worth" arguing about, like the upbringing of the children, finances, and sex. It is best in such situations to keep a cool head. This is good during arguments, helping you keep things in perspective – above all, it's good for one's health. Professor Robert Leverson of the renowned University of California at Berkeley tested 700 married couples. He put the couples into two categories: "cool" and "hot" conflict situations. While letting them talk about personal things he measured their blood pressure, pulse, and breathing rhythm.

> *Couples who can argue in a "cool" and objective fashion run less risk of ruining their relationship.*

The probability of couples splitting up within five years was much higher among the "hot" couples than the "cool." The "cool" couples discussed their problems quietly and from practical standpoints. The reason for this: The "heated" discussions were considered so disagreeable that the partners felt an "inner denial" and only wanted to get out of the discussion as soon as possible – even if that meant the problem was left unresolved.

An unexpected finding of the study was the difference between the sexes. Men can only tolerate extremely negative views for a relatively short period of time and they react with greater aversion to unpleasant situations. Women, on the other hand, were able to "deal" with the conflict longer. Apparently women do not experience such intense psychological side-effects in a conflict situation. Perhaps another bit of evidence of why heart attacks still (mainly) befall men?

Barnard Tips for a Healthy Heart

How You Can Best Cope with Your Feelings

1 **Don't take everything so seriously.**
   In a week's time you will probably laugh or have forgotten about many of the things that are upsetting you now.

2 **Talking brings relief.**
   Don't always deny yourself the comfort of sharing your problems. Tell someone about them.

3 **Don't be an egoist.**
   Of course everyone prefers to do the talking. But sometimes one has to shut up and listen.

4 **Be an egoist.**
   Don't hold back too much. Otherwise you will soon find yourself at the end of the line.

5 **Let off steam.**
   Ambition is important in life. But hopefully it isn't your only positive attribute.

6 **Think positive.**
   Agree with your partner on a sort of "thermostat of the emotions": if arguments must occur, they should be allowed to reach a certain point but no further.

7 **Give others a chance.**
   Of course you can do everything better. But if you never give others a chance to try, nobody will ever know it.

8 **Be honest.**
   Face your problems. You will see: we all have the same problems anyway.

9 **Become independent.**
   Of course your parents should be proud of you. But you should achieve your successes by yourself.

10 **Be human.**
   Even Arnold Schwarzenegger has been known to cry now and then.

Ambition is important in life. But hopefully it isn't your only positive attribute.

42 Keep Laughing

Take humor seriously. Laugh at your
reflection in the mirror every morning.
You will see it laugh back at you.

There is much wisdom in language – wisdom which for many could provide the right access to a healthy, enjoyable life. How little we pay attention to this fact! Even more astounding is our disregard of the golden rule, which for centuries has been part of the vernacular and which we seem to ignore almost completely: we have all heard the proverb "Laughter is the best medicine" since earliest childhood. But despite this, medical science has up until recently tended to ignore these words of wisdom. Only during the last decade of the last millennium did medicine take it upon itself to examine the effects of laughing. Only now is humor gaining the scientific acknowledgement that it has long deserved.

Strange as it might seem, a part of this delayed recognition was provided by Hollywood. The movie *Patch Adams* (1998), for example, depicts the major problems the real-life doctor Patch Adams had trying to convince the medical establishment of the many positive effects his "Clown Doctor" therapy had on children. Today this "clown doctor" is director of an institute in the state of Virginia and his theories are receiving recognition from all parts of the world.

How Hollywood made an international hit out of a simple idea.

But in the past things had not worked out like this. Until the time when Hollywood began to show an interest in this doctor and his "crazy" ideas, Adams' therapy had not been taken seriously by other doctors at all. But then everything happened very fast: laughter and healing did seem to have a reciprocal effect. This seemed reason enough for Hollywood to get in on the act – albeit a bit melodramatically. The time was ripe for Robin Williams to play the lead. The film was a success, as was laughter therapy soon afterwards.

The facts, as Patch Adams puts them, are quite simple. What has been called psychoneuroimmunology one could also call holistic medicine, based on the premise that the psychological and physical aspects of a case have to be taken equally seriously.

We have already seen that every form of stress – mental, spiritual, and physical – cause physiological and biochemical processes to take place in our bodies.

Among the many investigations of this topic, which – viewed scientifically – is still a relatively young and little-explored field, there has been clear agreement about one thing. Feelings like love, amazement, curiosity, passion, or joy, to mention just a few, serve to activate our immune system. In this way we stimulate the antibodies which make it difficult for all sorts of infections to attack our bodies. These positive feelings influence our heart too.

> *If you suppress your emotions, you are obstructing your body in its fight against illness.*

The Adams Idea

Negative feelings such as anger, aggression, loathing, and fury tend to "overwrite" our immune system. You can prevent this by overcoming these feelings – by allowing them to come out. If you give free rein to your emotions you will prevent the "bad feelings" from obstructing the antibodies. This is what Patch Adams was trying to say. And I must admit I am absolutely convinced that he is right.

Hollywood, by the way, is interested in me too. Years ago a film producer bought the film rights to my life story. The script writer and producer visited South Africa and, after a lengthy discussion, we agreed that the proposed film should not deal with my life but rather concentrate on the first human-to-human heart transplant, with only flashbacks of my life inserted here and there.

> *Laughter can prevent infection, cancer, and heart disease.*

But let's get back to laughter. I am very happy that "clinic clowns" and humor therapy are no longer treated like outsider methods in hospitals. Luckily science has recently found evidence to confirm the positive effects of laughter on patients and it can therefore be considered a form of therapy. The German psychologist Michael Titze points to the conclusions he has reached in various relevant studies. In one he found that a test group who laughed 20 minutes a day had a noticeably lower level of stress hormones in their blood.

It's Better to Laugh Out Loud

Titze, who has authored a series of books on therapeutic humor, is of the opinion that the preventive effect of laughter is most effective when it is supported phonetically – that is, he concludes that loud laughter is the best because it produces the most endorphins. These are the so-called "happiness hormones" which have a very positive effect on one's mood. As well as soothing pain, they help one to relax, give air to the lungs, and stimulate the immune system.

Studies at pediatric hospitals in the U.S. have shown that children in a "humorous" environment get well faster than those being treated in more sobering institutions. Today Patch Adams has become a kind of role model even though his methods were considered controversial and frowned upon by the medical establishment. His battles against the authorities and his superiors in the 1980s are legendary, but in the meantime an increasing number of hospitals are training doctors to go about their work with more humor. And you may not believe this, but now we even have a "world day of laughter."

I believe in the cleansing effect of humor. This has validity for heart attack prevention as well as for the preliminary stages of heart problems which are frequently a result of the demands our performance-oriented society puts on us. A person not able to keep up the pace in the workplace is immediately in danger of being the subject of ridicule and malice. This leads to his feeling offended and hurt, which then turns into shame, fear of failure, and increased tension. However, a person who resolves to include an ample share of laughter per day is able to deal with the effects of outside pressures. He no longer takes criticism to heart and is more relaxed because his own personal "laughter therapy" helps him to deal with performance pressure. Laughing about these things is the best thing you can do for your heart.

How many of you will be asking "Just how often a day should I laugh? What's good for the body and what isn't?" According to the latest scientific findings, most adults laugh about 20 times a day. But all laughter is not equal. An American study proved that for every 20 laughs, only four were "real." The others were expressions of politeness such as cordial chuckles when a friend or colleague says something mildly amusing.

> *Most people laugh about 20 times a day ...*

I would like to give you a personal tip pertaining to laughing. It's certainly harmless and can only help: laugh into the mirror every morning.

The World Wants to Be Amused

Increasingly often it is not only our reflection that smiles at us but the TV. The biggest private TV networks in Europe have apparently rediscovered just the thing to raise ratings: comedy. It's logical: as daily life becomes more frustrating for many of us, we look for diversion preferably of a light-hearted sort. Recently more and more comedy formats are making their appearance on our screens. Once again it was market research that convinced the network bosses that comedy would bring success. In a series of studies, British sociologist Oliver James concluded that the whole world has a craving for humor. James analyzed the data of 39,000 people from eight different countries and came to the conclusion that the likelihood of depression is three times higher today than 50 years ago.

> *... but only four of those are "real laughs."*

Does this mean that the great humor offensive has been launched? One could almost think so. The TV brings us more and more comedy programs and entertainment productions that aim to amuse us. There are also comedy clubs sprouting up all over. In Germany there are now 22 "laugh clubs," with 350 members who try to outdo each other in the laughter stakes. The entrepreneur Michael Berger conceived the idea of "laugh clubs" in the late 1990s, after he had read a statistic that Germans laugh only six minutes a day.

Germany organizes its humor with serious thoroughness. Laugh club members meet once a week in order to collectively burst out laughing. Nobody wears a false nose, no one tells any jokes. The 20-minute sessions begin with the participants standing in a circle clapping their hands and shouting "Ho-ho-ha-ha-ha." What then follows is a strictly regulated program of mirth in which the participants learn to laugh again.

The British intend to go a step further: they want to make laughter therapy available on prescription. A study revealed that people in 1990s Britain suffered 10 times more often from depressive ailments as in the 1950s. So the then-Minister for Health, Frank Dobson, made about £330 million of lottery money available for laughter therapy.

Patch Adams lent his personal support to this British initiative, and not only by giving speeches in a clown suit. The typically British dark sense of humor greeted the antics of Patch Adams with roars of laughter when he, dressed as an angel and carrying a harp, visited terminally ill patients or AIDS clinics and introduced himself as "the coming attraction." The British government expects the new laughter clinics to have a recognizable effect on the number of sick days lost to business every year.

Incredible but true: in the near future, comedians, magicians, and acrobats will be available in the U.K. on prescription. The doctor will determine the dosage, but generally it will probably be between 30 and 60 minutes' worth.

I think this will prove money well spent by the National Health Service, as the causal relationship between laughter and health is constantly being substantiated. It runs as follows: laughing slows the pulse and increases the flow of oxygen to the muscles. Endorphins – peptides produced by the body, creating an almost opium-like effect – stimulate a sense of well-being and are helpful in reducing stress.

Laughter Heals

Healing through humor, episode 1. How Norman Cousins "laughed" a life-threatening infection away.

Thirty years ago Norman Cousins contracted spondylarthritis, a painful, life-threatening inflammation of the spinal column. He was told by doctors that he would not have long to live and that the remaining time would be filled with almost intolerable pain. Cousins was convinced that pessimism had a negative effect on one's condition and the immune system. So he thought about how he could best counter this. He created for himself a "laugh system" which consisted of humorous books and films.

A miracle happened. After a period of time his pain subsided and soon after that he was diagnosed as completely cured. Doctors were puzzled about the reasons behind the strange but successful treatment: laughter and the positive attitude to life which it engenders.

Healing through humor, episode 2. How a Hollywood agent speeded up his cure by laughing.

The renowned Hollywood agent Paul Kohner told me about an unusual experience he had many decades ago. In the 1920s when he was still a young man and before he emigrated from Germany to the United States with the mighty film tycoon Carl Laemmle, and there befriended and looked after luminaries like Albert Einstein, Ingrid Bergman, John Huston, and Ernest Hemingway (to name but a few) he had to undergo an appendix operation.

Shortly after the operation a fellow patient lying in the bed next to him had acted the clown, "becoming funnier and funnier. I thought my stitches would burst."

The result? The scar healed well and Kohner was able to leave the hospital much sooner than the doctors had anticipated.

Just two of many examples taken from everyday life which show that humor is good for one's health. Almost all the other scientific explanations concerning the positive effects of laughter are of more recent origin. An example: the biochemist L. S. Berk proved only as recently as the 1990s that the so-called "killer cells" which serve the immune system are activated by laughter.

It's astounding what a heartfelt laugh can accomplish: it increases the production of immunoglobulin in the saliva and in the blood. It also increases the cytokine *gamma-interferon*, which inhibits the increase of tumor cells and which has recently been making headlines in cancer research.

> *100 peals of laughter are as valuable as 10 minutes' training on a rowing machine.*

A person who laughs a lot protects his or her heart from infections which could lead to cardiac arrest. Hearty laughter increases the production of hormones. Laughing literally refreshes the heart: it has the same effect on our body as sport. Researchers at Stanford University have found the 100 peals of laughter can have the same effect as 10 minutes' training on a rowing machine.

The Center of Laughter

How does laughter actually work? Scientists from the University of Southern California in Los Angeles discovered, mostly by chance, the organic root of our laughter. They were in the process of examining a young girl who suffered from epilepsy. They stimulated approximately 100 points on her frontal brain lobes with weak electric shocks. When they stimulated an approximately 2-square-inch area on the upper part of the lobes, she started laughing. It appears certain that this small area in our brain, located very close to our speech center, is responsible for our "sense" of humor.

> *Until recently, scientists used to poke fun at laughter as therapy. Now it has become a science of its own.*

In the meantime science no longer relies on chance. Just recently an independent field of research has evolved called gelotology, which comes from the Greek word *gelos* (laughter). Gelotologists – researchers in the science of laughter – are attempting to answer the many still-open questions concerning laughter and the connection between mental and physical well-being. From a medicinal point of view I think that we will be hearing a lot more about laughter in the years to come. But I can already urge you to take humor to heart. Try to determine whether laughter is not in fact your best everyday medication. Find ways of laughing at work. That will help to relax the muscles of your face. Even if you don't feel like laughing, your cheerful face will at least give pleasure to those around you.

Barnard Tips for a Healthy Heart
Why You Must Try to Laugh

1 **More success**
   Cheerful people are better able to cope with job stress.
2 **More sex appeal**
   Laughing is sexy. This goes for men too.
3 **More oxygen**
   Laughing works like an oxygen mask. Four times as much oxygen enters the body when we are laughing.
4 **More fitness**
   Laughing has the same effect as jogging or swimming.
5 **More relaxation**
   Laughing reduces the stress hormones.
6 **More resistance**
   Laughing stimulates the immune system.
7 **More friends**
   There are reasons for the saying "laughter is contagious."
8 **More money**
   Perhaps laughter will save you from expensive psychotherapy.

9 More health

Scientifically proven: illnesses can be laughed away.

10 More fun

Last but not least: laughing makes life more fun.

43 Don't Hide Grief

Grief can be dangerous – but helpful
too. Read here why this need not be
a contradiction in terms.

From my experience as a physician and from my personal
experience, I know that grief, sorrow, and mourning are essential
components of our lives. Practically all relevant psychological
studies refer to the usefulness of so-called "sorrow work" (dealing
with sadness in our lives). A person who neglects to deal with
sorrow or suppresses it will probably have to deal with the consequences later on.

I say this fully aware of the fact that some medical studies have
also warned of the dangers of sorrow. For instance, immediately
after the death of a loved one – be it a person or pet – the risk of a
heart attack is particularly high.

An American study done over a four-year time span questioned
1,774 people in the week after they'd suffered a heart attack.
Among the questions asked was whether any grave misfortune
had befallen them just before the attack. More than 200 of the test
group answered yes! The scientists concluded that immediately
after the death of a spouse, parent or child, the heart attack risk is
14 times the average!

Boston University professor Murray Mittleman has focused his
efforts on studies of stress as a result of sorrow. However, he
admits, "Scientifically the theory that emotional stress can trigger
a cardiac arrest cannot be completely confirmed." It's possible

that mental anguish can, for rather obvious reasons, increase the risk of a heart attack. One is a biological factor, the other more "human":

1 Sorrow sends our hormone levels spiralling upwards.
2 Due to the general confusion brought about by the feelings of sorrow, mourners frequently lose their appetite, suffer from lack of sleep, and even forget to take medication that they desperately need.

As I've said, I think it is absolutely necessary that people be allowed to express their sorrow. I personally have experienced three very strong periods of sorrow in my life. One after the death of my eldest son, then when my charismatic father died suddenly and unexpectedly, and finally after the death of my second wife Barbara, even though we had been divorced for many years.

The renowned Viennese psychiatrist Erwin Ringel once said that dealing with grief is very important for the soul. I think that he was quite correct.

One of My Most Sorrowful Experiences

I once experienced a form of emotional stress which I haven't been able to get rid of to this day. An African boy of about 10 years old was brought to me in Cape Town with a severe cardiac failure brought about by rheumatic fever.

One of his heart valves was completely destroyed and leaking severely; to make matters worse he still suffered from rheumatic inflammation of the heart muscle. Under ordinary circumstances we would have delayed the operation to allow the inflammation of the heart muscle to subside, but as he was so sick we were forced to replace the valve that night.

The operation was completed without much difficulty and the patient was transferred to the intensive care unit. The next morning when I visited him, I was shocked to note that his condition had deteriorated. After increasing the medication to improve a pumping action of his heart, without response, I realized that he was dying. Not knowing what further to do, I put my head under the oxygen tent and asked him whether there was anything else he wanted. His answer was, "A piece of bread." He died clutching the piece of bread in his little hand as if it were his most valuable possession.

This experience has stayed with me and fills me with sadness even today, because I know that if he had had enough bread earlier on in his short life he probably would not have developed rheumatic fever.

The death of a loved one is not the only grief we experience in our lives. We are subjected to many other kinds of traumatic experience. The sorrows of love affairs gone wrong, arguments with parents, yes, even trivial things like when our favorite team loses a football match can engender deep sadness. We must learn to cope with all forms of sorrow, great or small. We must not bury our head in the sand. Face reality – as difficult as that may be. That is the advice I would like to give you for every form of sorrow.

Barnard Tips for a Healthy Heart

Overcoming the Pangs of Love

1 **Eat what you like.**
  Many people find chocolate comforting when they're feeling down.
2 **Try spring cleaning.**
  Let the vacuum cleaner help you overcome. It may knock the photo of your ex-partner off the mantle piece – accidentally, of course.
3 **Spoil yourself.**
  Take yourself to the movies – even if nobody else does.
4 **Go shopping.**
  Not a bad idea at all – as long as your credit card can take it.
5 **Do sport.**
  Run your heart out – not literally, of course.
6 **Make plans.**
  Think ahead to the time when you will have overcome your heartache.
7 **Be honest.**
  No glorifying post-mortem: he/she wasn't as fantastic as all that.

8 **Make contacts.**

Renew old friendships.

9 **Analyze it.**

No excuses. Why did your relationship really fail?

10 **Flirt away.**

There's nothing like a bit of harmless flirting to boost your self-confidence.

44 Learn to Manage Your Anger

Continuous anger obstructs the immune
system in its work – the prevention of
cancer and heart attack.

It's Monday morning and somehow nothing seems go right. You are late, the children are grumbling, and your wife chooses this time to discuss some function she is planning for next weekend. The car takes a long time to start, then you go and land in a major traffic jam. Your boss is upset because you're late (why do bosses never seem to get caught up in traffic jams?). In the course of the morning a particularly unpleasant client phones you. At lunch a tooth caves in. Unfortunately your dentist is on holiday and her stand-in has a waiting list of two weeks.

> *Try to keep calm. That will help your heart and improve your career prospects.*

There are occasions in life where one could go mad. I can only advise you: don't do it. Anger is an inevitable part of life. If you remember that, you will regain your composure more quickly and more easily.

By this I am not recommending that you swallow everything. Not by a long chalk. But of what use is it to shout at your children, cut your wife short, and signal behind your boss's back what you think of him? After all, there's at least one Monday in every week.

It's better to be prepared. Get ready for the next unpleasant situation. Begin by taking stock – what kind of person are you? Do you lose your temper easily? Do you always give vent to your anger regardless of the consequences? If you answered all these questions "yes," then you are part of a very high-risk group, because people who get angry – and stay that way – often raise their heart attack risk greatly.

Be honest and ask yourself: what did I get upset about these last weeks, and of what real importance were the issues that upset me? Such questions asked in retrospect will probably cause you to smile weakly about much that incensed you. Much of it wasn't worth getting so excited about, was it?

So keep a cool head. That's a characteristic much in demand today anyway. Or do you think that your boss will entrust a hot-head with an important task?

"Keep a cool head" – why do we say that? Well, anger really gets your body going. The blood gets thicker, the arteries narrow, your blood pressure rises and the heart pumps faster. On the outside this can be seen in an angry person's red face. If you can control your anger, you can stay "cool." "That's very difficult," you might say. It isn't. Carl Thoresen, a doctor at the famous Stanford University in California, specializes in anger management. He recommends three behavior patterns when it comes to managing situations that generate anger:

1 Change your anger!
2 Avoid your anger!
3 Adapt to your anger!

However, don't suppress your anger either, I'd like to add here. I'll give you a practical example from my life. A short time ago I came across an article in a European tabloid about my wife filing for divorce. The story was filled with lies about me, my wife, and the reasons we were getting a divorce. Still, I did not let the article make me angry.

> *A quick way to avoid too much anger in your life.*

Had I let it irritate me then I would have been upset, but what would that have achieved? Nothing but endangering my heart.

I reacted with composure to the story, in accordance with the third point of Dr. Thoresen's three recommendations. I could have chosen point 2 and ignored the story completely, or even point 1 and found a way to channel my anger.

Perhaps in a way I did do that as well – because my first reaction was laughter – the story was so ridiculous. But the serious fact is that anger can take up so much of our lives if we let it. Since more and more people find themselves unable to cope with negative feelings such as anger and rage, courses and clinics have been established throughout the world to help people learn how to deal better with their anger. The results have not only been encouraging, they have provided new insights and discoveries into the phenomenon of anger.

DISCOVERY NO. 1: ASPIRIN HELPS

Murray Mittleman, director of the American Institute for Heart, Lung and Blood Diseases, and his colleague James E. Muller found evidence that their "anger patients" had a 230% higher cardiac arrest risk after an emotional experience than patients who did not react with anger to the emotional experience. In the course of this study they discovered that aspirin had a powerful effect on the "anger patients." Those who took an aspirin daily had a 50% lower incidence of cardiac arrest. The reason: aspirin thins the blood, thereby reducing the development of the small blood clots which can block an artery and lead to a heart attack.

> *A person who often gets excited runs a greater risk of having a heart attack.*

DISCOVERY NO. 2: NUTRITION HELPS

I also believe that a person's diet plays an important role in anger and aggression. This opinion is supported by a study I heard about many years ago. It was researched by a psychologist at Stony Brook University in New York State. He investigated the eating patterns of 233 families in the state of Oregon. Particularly interesting was the fact that the families who took care to eat a low-fat diet had a completely different behavior pattern to those who ate "normally." The "diet families" had a much lower incidence of hostility and aggression than the others did.

DISCOVERY NO. 3: ADVICE HELPS

Heart patients in California who agreed to receive counseling along with their traditional medical treatment had a 60% better success ratio than patients who did not partake in the counseling sessions. Similar results were achieved in studies carried out at Stanford University. The patients of the most common anger type (constantly moving about, aggressive, and hostile) who had learned to deal more effectively with their emotions had a much better chance of avoiding a second heart attack than their fellow patients who did not undergo "stress management." Fifty percent fewer suffered a second cardiac arrest.

Professor Ichiro Kawachi of Harvard University made an even more dramatic observation in a study undertaken over the course of seven years involving 1,300 men. The men, with an average age of 62, were put in categories according to anger potential. The end result was astounding. Those with the highest anger/emotional levels clearly had the highest number of heart attacks – three times higher than those with the lowest levels.

By the way, the most common type of "anger patients" – described by scientists as angry, mean, and distant – were also examined according to their genetic make-up. It was established that they had a higher level of adrenaline and more stress hormones in their bloodstream.

So let us reiterate: a low-fat diet, an aspirin per day – provided you don't have a gastric ulcer! – and approximately one year of therapy by an expert who can provide advice for dealing with anger will heal everyone – and particularly the inherent and the habitual "anger types." A major step in the prevention of heart attacks could be taken if these tips were followed by those in danger!

45 | Be Honest

20 times a day, our noses makes
Pinocchios of us. Stop lying, you're
damaging your heart.

You probably don't admit this even to yourself, but it's true: there is a liar in all of us. Sociological studies have proven that the average person lies between 15 and 20 times a day. We are not talking here of unfaithful husbands who are constantly having to be "economical" with the truth. The lies referred to here are mostly little, social ones – for instance when we answer the question "How are you?" with "Fine, thanks" even though we feel terrible. Or when we describe our last holiday in glowing terms when in fact we really couldn't wait to get back home again.

> *The most common lies: "I'm very well, thanks" and "I've stopped smoking."*

Lying is a strange thing. It has become a part of our everyday lives. Through fibbing we avoid unpleasant situations, keep our social and love lives in good order, and create time for ourselves. "I'm sorry, I can't come to work today, I've got a sore throat." "But darling, I simply forgot you don't like strawberry ice cream." "We're terribly sorry, we can't make it to your party. The dog has sprained her foot." Nowhere else in life are we as creative as in the thinking up of lies and excuses.

Men and women are equally adept at lying. Bella DePaulo, professor of psychology at the University of Virginia, found no gender differences in this respect. In a conversation lasting 10 minutes, we lie for two of those minutes. Twenty years ago a study at the University of Bath in England had found that men lie 10 times as often as women. By 10 years ago it had become three times as often. And now: "Women lie every bit as well as men," says the German psychologist Birgit Mentzen.

Lying, particularly at the office, is part of trying to impress. As more and more women enter and remain in the workforce, they resort to exaggerations, excuses, and little white lies more frequently.

> *Women have learned to lie as well as men ...*

Professor DePaulo also found that educated people are more successful liars. She tested 2,000 people from various social strata. The result: students and university graduates lie best. Their linguistic ability and their self-confidence make them great manipulators with words.

> *... but the best liars are students and university graduates.*

Yet it's so important not to lie, believe me. Above all one should not lie to the person with whom one should be most honest – oneself. This honesty is critical to our health. Test yourself. Do you always correctly give your weight? Do you lie to yourself about your eating habits? Those few excess pounds, those hours of sitting in front of a computer, just a couple of cigarettes: they're not worth mentioning, even to yourself. Really? Have you looked at yourself in the mirror lately? Hasn't your nose grown just a little?

That story about Pinocchio is actually nearer the truth than we might like to believe. When we are untruthful, blood collects in our nose. This mini-swelling cannot be seen with the naked eye, but it is measurable. Dr. Alan Hirsch, chairperson of the Smell and Taste Foundation in Chicago, maintains that we can expose liars by watching their noses. They tend to raise a hand to their nose much more often than usual. His best recent example: Bill Clinton. In cooperation with his colleague, Charles Wolf of the University of Illinois, Hirsch analyzed the video of Clinton's testimony in the

Monica Lewinsky inquiry. In the course of the examination the American president tended to want to touch his nose more and more.

The first step on the road to greater health calls for greater honesty. Here are the 10 "everyday" lies you should consign to the dustbin:

LIE 1: I'M NOT REALLY A SMOKER

You never buy cigarettes, and if someone asks you whether you smoke, you deny it vehemently. But if you were to count every single one, how many did you have last week – 10, 20, 50, 100?

Stop it. See yourself as a smoker and begin to drop the habit. Not next week or after the holidays. You must begin today!

LIE 2: I'M REALLY QUITE FIT

You know all about the new running shoes and you've never missed a Formula One Grand Prix on TV. But does that really make you a sportsman? Movement and activity is something no one can do for you. You must get up and do it yourself, better now than later. Regardless of your age group – 17 or 70 – even a 15-minute walk or climbing the stairs instead of taking the elevator helps you become fit and builds up resistance against illness. Remember, you can always video-record the Grand Prix and watch it after your workout.

LIE 3: I'M NOT STRESSED

You work more than 10 hours a day, and on top of that you bring home piles of documents. Not a good idea. Apart from the fact that your partner will soon think you are no longer interested in your relationship (a fact your workload may prevent you from realizing at all!), you are depriving your body of its most important form of relaxation. Your evenings and weekends belong to your family and to your body. No one is irreplaceable; not everyone has to do it all. Learn to delegate. After all, they only pay you one salary.

LIE 4: I'M NOT REALLY OVERWEIGHT

Of course you can pass through a door sideways if you find it too difficult to do so head-on. But perhaps it is time to be honest with yourself. You have put on quite a lot and you will have to lose a few pounds. You will probably not have to diet. Just eat less. For a few days this will not be so easy, but you'll see: after a week at most you will no longer be as painfully aware of the fact that you are eating only as much as you need.

LIE 5: I'M NOT REALLY AN UNHEALTHY EATER

You know about vegetables because you drive past a vegetable market every day. Fruit makes a wonderful table decoration. This won't do. Both of these food groups belong on your plate – several times a day. You don't like vegetables? No problem. Try using herbs and spices so that you don't even taste the vegetables. Or try vegetable juice for a change.

LIE 6: I'M QUITE CAPABLE OF RELAXING

When you come home in the evening, do you first kiss your wife and then look for the TV remote control? And do you fall asleep after two hours in front of the boob tube? Perhaps you even think of this as a good way to relax? It isn't. Movement in the fresh air, reading, meeting friends, being active – these things clear your head.

LIE 7: I DON'T NEED TO BE CHOOSY ABOUT MY DOCTOR

You choose your mechanic, plumber, or insurance agent very carefully. But you choose your doctor based on who's nearest. Your doctor can play a very important role in your life. Of course you spend more time in your car than at the doctor's. But when your car breaks down for good, you can buy a new one. Try doing that with your body.

LIE 8: I KNOW ABOUT THESE THINGS

You subscribe to five current affairs magazines and with your satellite dish you can receive at least 50 TV channels. So you are really at the hub of things. Wonderful. But when your children come home from school with an assignment, you are the first to look for an excuse not to help so as not to make a fool of yourself. Be honest and don't be afraid of asking "dumb questions" – and this goes for your health as well. Don't be afraid to ask your doctor to cut through all the jargon. None of us knows everything; in actual fact we all know damn little.

LIE 9: NOBODY PULLS THE WOOL OVER MY EYES

You think of yourself as a mature consumer, and advertising does not influence you one bit. But when a new type of mobile phone comes on the market, you can't wait to buy it. You should continue to be skeptical, particularly as far as your health is concerned. An increasing number of "foreign" branches are getting involved in the health business. The "product" they provide is very often incomplete, imprecise or completely wrong. So be sure to inform yourself about the source from which you acquire your knowledge. Many charlatans have become rich at the expense, pain, and agony of countless families.

LIE 10: I'M HONEST WITH MYSELF

You have read the above and in most cases you have decided that these lies do not apply to you. I suggest you read them once more and try to be really honest with yourself. Or: let your partner assess you for a change. You will be surprised at what others think of you. Believe me: the sooner you realize that you are not perfect either, the sooner you will be able to do something good for your heart.

46 Make Friends

Sociable people are ill less often.
The "feel good" factor is becoming
ever more important in our society.

Isolation has become a national disease. It affects more and more people, causing ever-increasing suffering. Socially isolated people are more susceptible to infectious diseases and run a higher risk of developing heart problems. The 21st century is becoming the era of the pensioner. The over-60 age group is growing all the time. If the trend continues, the social integration of lonely people will become one of the big challenges.

I am afraid that this is going to get even worse over the course of time. The youth culture that dominates advertising and the media, the increasing pace of life – which overtaxes more and more people, particularly the aged – these things are going to have to change. If society doesn't start with a counter-movement in time, then we will be confronted by a serious divide between the under-50s and over-50s.

> *Lonely people run a greater risk of cardiac arrest.*

Early studies tended to point to the fact that it was mostly men who had difficulty dealing with the phenomenon of isolation and as a result suffered more from heart ailments. However, more recent studies show that isolation is no longer gender-specific.

In Sweden a study was recently made public that examined a group of 300 people. They all were women between 30 and 65 who had one thing in common: social isolation.

The researchers from the Karolinska Hospital and the Royal Institute of Stockholm were investigating the so-called HRV (Heart Rate Viability) among women. Heart Rate Viability is a kind of "spy" that provides information concerning a person's ability to cope with daily stress. The study showed that these isolated women had much more difficulty coping with stress than 300 comparable women with social contacts.

A person who has neither friends nor relatives runs twice as great a risk of becoming ill.

An interesting study was undertaken by the Carnegie-Mellon University in Pittsburgh. Sheldon Cohen, a psychologist at the university, studied 276 volunteers, men and women between the ages of 18 and 55. They were exposed to a cold virus – but first they were asked to fill out a questionnaire through which their social contacts could be analyzed: how many friends they had, if they belonged to any organizations or groups, contact with their family, and so on. One thing can be said straight away: the stronger the social network, the less likely the person was actually to contract the virus. Individuals involved in fewer than three social groups contracted the virus twice as frequently as those who had up to six different social contacts. Because the observations were made during different times of the year, it is safe to say that the results were not in any way influenced by the seasons. Neither were they influenced by age, gender, nationality, or education.

Cohen calls this phenomenon the "feel good" factor, which provides the body with increased defenses against viral infections. The more recognition people receive in their social environment, the more positive their mood, which then affects their hormonal balance and the release of the body's "disease killers." Cohen is still not sure how the psychological effect turns into a physiological one. He will try and determine this in his next study.

He has, however, found a similar behavior pattern in the

animal kingdom. Monkeys who are high up in the hierarchy of their group are less likely to get ill.

How I Landed in a New York Jail

Sociological studies have always interested me greatly. Whenever the opportunity arises I try to test any theories that I might have. One time I went to New York City to be named an "Honorary Fire Fighter" by the Mayor. After the ceremonies I was asked if I had any unfulfilled wish: whatever the mayor had the power to do would be done for me. To everyone's surprise, I asked to visit a jail.

My request was granted and I was able to spend some time with the inmates, who were first offenders. They were divided into discussion groups, and one of the topics particularly interested me: "A man alone is in bad company." I could only agree, knowing as I do that people who have difficulty dealing with daily stress situations and who lack social contacts place their heart and general health in serious danger. To put it another way: lonely people die younger.

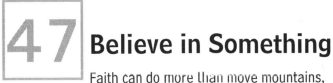

47 Believe in Something

Faith can do more than move mountains,
it can prolong your life. There is increasing
proof of this.

I believe in the healing power of positive thoughts. I know that many of my international colleagues agree with me on this subject. A heart surgeon from Vienna, Professor Ernst Wollner, whom I know very well and whose work I admire a great deal, told me once, "I have great difficulty with patients who are fearful and negative before an operation." I can understand him very well. During the thousands of operations I performed in my career, those patients who had the greatest chance of survival were those who believed in the success of the procedure.

> *Pessimism is the worst medicine.*

I have a firm belief in God and I used to say a prayer before every operation. That helped me when I stood in the operating theatre. I simply never felt alone. And yet it was important each time that the patient was also in a positive frame of mind. I have heard people say before an operation: "I believe I will soon be dead." And although they came successfully through the worst, these people often died soon afterward. Perhaps they had simply lost the will to live.

In the latter part of my career I was hesitant to operate on people who insisted that they would not recover from the operation.

I seriously believed that this negative attitude interfered with their recovery. Healing takes effort. If you don't have the will to fight an illness, you stand much less chance of becoming healthy again.

Belief and a positive mental attitude are essential characteristics in the well-being of an individual. It is very lucky that these facts are today accepted by science.

The belief in a higher power, whatever that may be, not only gives life more meaning, it also improves one's overall physical condition and increases life expectancy. Just recently two American studies were able to provide decisive evidence for this claim.

If you don't believe in yourself, you literally get less out of life.

In the so-called land of opportunity, the U.S., there is a wealth of TV evangelists. A few of these have been unmasked as greedy profiteers who worshipped only the almighty dollar. But this has not changed the fact that these "pastors" are still about, peddling their form of religion to unsuspecting "wanna believers." Apparently there is a market that the traditional religions do not reach. As I said at the beginning of this chapter, people seem to need something that they can cling to.

If they can't find it through priests, doctors or – the best solution – within themselves, then they may turn to charlatans.

How can belief and religion lengthen life expectancy? This is a case the researchers are still not quite sure of. Up until now it has been purely speculation why people going to church services are generally healthier. The feeling of belonging, it has been said, strengthens the immune system.

- Belief can lengthen your life.
- Those who attend church once or more a week live, on average, eight years longer than "non-believers." The difference in age reached is also convincing – 75 years for the non-believers and 83 years for the faithful. The data for this study was based mostly on information provided by the American Institute of National Health.
- Belief keeps you healthy.

- A further, highly praised example is a study done by J. LeBron McBride of the Baptist Hospital in Morrow, Georgia. He examined 442 religious patients according to the success of their treatment and sensitivity to pain. According to the results, the "believers" were healthier and had a higher pain threshold. LeBron McBride even went so far as to recommend that doctors should enquire about patients' religious beliefs during the initial consultation
  I can certainly imagine how the answer to the question, "Do you believe in a higher power?" would make a difference in a doctor's approach to dealing with an individual's health problems.

Douglas Oman and Dwayne Reed are two doctors who have already asked patients this question. The two worked for five years on a study at the Buck Center Clinic in Novato, California, which deals exclusively with geriatric research. Approximately 2,000 volunteers, none younger than 55, were asked how often they attended church.

They also asked basic questions about habits, mental health, physical fitness, and social contact. After five years, 24% more of the test group who regularly attended church service were still alive. This 24% was an absolute statistic after other risk factors such as age, sex habits, mental health, and other aspects had been considered.

> *Faith doesn't only move mountains – it also supports your immune system.*

The researchers concluded that the connection between health and religion could not be overlooked, but nor should it be viewed as anything other than a complementary factor. Religious belief can be seen as part of a basically positive outlook on life.

What is belief for most of us? A way of making sense of life. A goal to aim for. Belief gives us hope. Optimism is one of the strongest powers that we can develop. Positive thinking and trust in one's own power not only help the soul. They promote good health as well.

A group of scientists from the University of California, led by immunologist John Fahey and psychologist Susan Segerstrom, examined people who were under extreme mental strain. Ninety law students at University of California at Los Angeles volunteered for the study. The group was between 20 and 37 years old. Nine in the group were married and had families.

Fahey, Segerstrom, and their team examined the blood samples of these students to check the number of immune cells such as B-cells, T-killer cells, and T-helper cells. At the same time, written tests were given to assess the students' state of mind, stress, and health awareness. The figures for the immune cells at the beginning of the study (which coincided with the first term of their law studies) were virtually identical for both groups. By the middle of the first term, when the procedure was repeated, the results differed. The immune cells of the "optimists" had risen significantly (on average about 13%) while those of the pessimists were down slightly. They had an average of 3% fewer immune cells in their blood. Clearly this is good evidence for the fact that health, optimism, confidence, and belief are very closely linked.

> *Optimism doesn't always come naturally, but one can learn it.*

The well-known German motivational expert Nikolaus B. Enkelmann says, "Every goal that I envisage, I can reach with the right attitude." It is often not the most able, ambitious, or best-educated people who succeed at university, are happy in their private lives, and do well in their profession. It is almost always the optimists. Believe in yourself and in life.

Barnard Tips for a Healthy Heart
Things to Believe In – If You Want to!

1 **Believe in God.**
   For some people the conventional way is still the best.
2 **Believe in yourself.**
   Don't wait for others to do it. Believe in yourself.
3 **Believe in the comet.**
   Perhaps it will come. But I wouldn't bet on it.
4 **Believe in life after death.**
   More important would be to know: is it better than this life?

5 **Believe in computer chaos.**

The 21st century might be the time to get back to basics.

6 **Believe in a better life.**

The optimist's favourite expression: "Everything is going to be all right."

7 **Believe in basic human goodness and decency.**

Perhaps if you look for it long enough ...

8 **Believe in the power of destiny.**

It's fate! So what can you do about it?

9 **Believe in nothing.**

This may eventually leave you much too empty.

10 **Believe in love.**

You should definitely give your heart this chance.

48 Do Some Rethinking

Nothing is more difficult than breaking
a habit. Think of some way to reward yourself.

Think a bit about the way you are presently living. You've been living in the same house for two decades. You've always driven the same type of car. And you've been married to the same person for 30 years now. You always buy your meat from the same butcher and spend all your holidays in Florida – in the same hotel. When the manager of that hotel retired two years ago, making way for a younger man, you saw this as an unwelcome disruption in the order of things.

Now imagine someone coming to you and saying, "This will all have to change. You will have to move, get a different car, and take your holidays in Jamaica instead of Florida." Don't think of this as madness, because it is exactly what I would recommend. If you have done nothing for your heart so far, then it is high time you do some – systematic rethinking.

Nothing is more difficult to change than the habits of a lifetime, even when they have been proven to have a very negative influence on our health. Smoking, obesity – as a result of eating too much or not exercising enough – and stress are the biggest risk factors. What they all have in common is that they are not circumstances we're born with. It is up to us to learn to eat healthily, to reduce the stress we subject ourselves to, to stop smoking once and for all.

If you want badly enough to do these things, take the first step now.

STEP 1: ANALYSIS

What does your life really look like? That is the first question you should try to answer. Ask yourself what factors in your life increase the risk of cardiovascular ailments, and draw your own conclusions from this. Sure, you are slightly overweight, one can see that. And you smoke, as all about you can smell. But are you also being honest about your stress levels? Real insight is the first step towards change. Only when you have fully accepted that your lifestyle up to now has been unhealthy in various ways, will you be ready to drop some ingrained habits.

STEP 2: THE REVELATION

So you are overweight and your cholesterol level is also too high. But there are at least eight other important heart-risk factors. Just two don't add up to anything really serious, right? Wrong. Having two risk factors may not only double but even quadruple the risk of a heart attack. If you are not only too heavy and have too much cholesterol, but are also completely inactive, your risk could be 16-fold. Already, your case has taken on a dramatic note.

> *You smoke, are overweight, and inactive: then your risk of heart attack is 16 times greater than average.*

STEP 3: THE PLAN

OK, you have become convinced that you must do something for your health. Think of something. Just saying, "I won't eat fat anymore" or "I'll lose a few pounds" is a bit weak. Devise specific, realistic goals for yourself – and think of how to reward yourself when you achieve them. No, I don't mean that you should fast for a week, then reward yourself with a meal lasting several hours! Show more subtlety. Try to define how you want to feel after changing your habits – when you weigh less, for instance, or have more efficient lungs. You will see: when you truly reach a goal you have set yourself, that in itself will be quite a reward.

You can take the most important steps to preventing heart problems all by yourself. Don't forget the simple things in life: a regular, written account of your blood pressure readings can provide your doctor with crucial information.

Take your pulse regularly. Don't be satisfied with measuring your blood pressure only when you're resting and at the same time every day. The ideal information can be gathered if it is taken a few times a day and after different activities. I've already showed you how your heart rate should increase during proper training. Just to recap, first you work out your maximum heart rate (220 minus your age). Your heart rate during sporting activity should always lie in the region of 50 to 75% of this maximum frequency. If you are 50, then your maximum heart rate is 170. The pulse rate you should aim at when training should, in this case, not exceed 127 beats per minute.

Just as important as your personal blood pressure statistic and finding your ideal pulse rate are regular visits to your doctor. Especially if you're healthy. What always surprises me is how many people neglect having a regular check-up. This is particularly true among men. For me it's incomprehensible that people put off their annual check-up or simply just "forget" it.

> *Every third man doesn't go to the doctor – even when he is experiencing the symptoms of an approaching heart attack.*

A survey done by an American health magazine and the news network CNN among 1,000 adults, unveiled a startling truth which was hard to believe in the apparently health-conscious United States. The survey showed that 37% of all the men questioned stated that they would not seek medical advice even if they experienced shortness of breath. A further 34% would not even seek a doctor's help if they experienced chest pains. Almost every child today knows that these are the first signs of an impending heart attack.

The explanation for this unbelievable ignorance, which in part could explain the high death rate from heart attacks in the U.S., could lie in a faulty value system. For many men, going to the doctor is still felt to be a sign of weakness. One does this only when one is really ill, not to prevent illness.

This is a potentially fatal misconception. Just think: 60% of patients feel absolutely nothing before their first heart attack. No warning at all. The attack takes them completely by surprise. This alone should be enough reason, even for those who feel healthy or who have not yet experienced any symptoms of coronary heart problems, to see their doctor at regular intervals.

The Wonder Weapons of Modern Medicine

Medicine has made great progress in recent times. The devices that modern medicine has available today are particularly effective for making early diagnoses. In the U.S. a device has been developed – the electronic-beam tomograph – which for me has only one disadvantage: it is extremely expensive. But it provides invaluable data by being able to edit pictures of the heart in intervals of 50 milliseconds. Because our heart, as I mentioned in my introduction, is but a primitive muscle whose only function is to pump, measuring its speed is more important for an exact examination than technically brilliant photography. The object is to catch the heart in that fraction of a second when it goes from the pump phase to the rest phase. Conventional computer tomographs (CTs) are bit too slow to accomplish this.

The electronic-beam CT does this effortlessly. With these pictures even the degree of calcium deposits can be ascertained. Calcium deposits in blood vessels are very important indicators of vascular disease.

But what use is the best and most expensive diagnostic instrument if nobody goes to the doctor?

49 | Program Your Brain

Use your brain like a computer.
Delete "unhealthy" data and replace
it with "healthy" information.

The human mind is a wonder of nature. It functions as well as any computer and it can be programmed like a computer. The data that you "save" in your "hard drive" dictates your lifestyle. If you want to change your lifestyle you must enter the relevant data, reprogramming your brain. Believe me, this works.

> *The computer program for your brain: delete – enter new info – save.*

Let us go on with this metaphor: imagine that your brain is like a second-hand computer you buy in a store. At home you set up the computer, switch it on – and find that its contents are in a state of chaos. Documents, programs, all mixed up. There is much there that you can't use, and other, important material that's missing. What will you do now?

- Clean your computer. Out goes everything you don't need. That saves space and improves your capabilities.
- Feed your computer – with all the new programs which you need for work and entertainment.
- Treat your computer well. Prepare it gently for its new tasks, only installing as much as it can comfortably take.

- Test your computer. When you have completed the installation, you do a test run. Is everything working? Is everything in place?

Treat your brain the same way. Reprogram it. Delete the data which is responsible for an unhealthy lifestyle. Feed your brain with everything that you want to do in a new way in your life. And then save this new data.

This has also been called the "change history method," and it is becoming increasingly popular. The reason is obvious: "changing history" works according to a simple principle, can be used by anyone, and has an enormously high success rate. You should make use of it.

Let us assume that you smoke. You've probably made a few attempts to quit. You've been unsuccessful every time because in your subconscious mind you are quite convinced that you cannot get by without cigarettes. Now try the "change history method." Do it as though you were using a video camera. All the "change history method" requires is that you "play" yourself the "film" of your last failure to stop smoking and, as it flickers across your mind, try and keep your composure. While in this calm mood, you just turn the event around and, in your mind, make it into a great success. After all, you did make it through two days without cigarettes. See yourself managing to live for two days without cigarettes. Wonderful. Store this as a positive achievement. For the first time in years you were able to breathe freely again. Excellent. You really managed that well ...

Repeat this procedure a few times until your last attempt to quit smoking has imprinted itself on your brain as a positive experience rather than a negative one.

Our central nervous system plays a vital role in the "change history method." The central nervous system simply relays stimuli – it does not determine whether these stimuli are real or imagined. So when the cue "stop smoking" is not associated with the stimulus of a defeat (the normal stimulus upon being unsuccessful), then the central nervous system may transport other signals which it has picked up to the brain: the cleaner breath which you had during your last attempt to give up smoking, the improved sense of taste, the greater sense of general well-being.

Basically four essential steps are necessary in order to program the computer in your mind successfully to make difficult changes such as quitting smoking, changing your eating habits, or making exercise part of your daily routine:

Step 1   Delete
          To be on the safe side, try and remember everything one
          more time before deleting it for good.
Step 2   Relax
          If you feel uncomfortable while you're mentally reviewing
          your past failures, then shake off this feeling with relaxation
          exercises, or keep interrupting the process until the
          negative side-effects have disappeared.
Step 3   Load
          Enter the "new script" and store it in your memory by
          repeating it many times.
Step 4   Believing it
          Believe what your inner computer is showing you. This
          conviction will help you – whatever you decide to do.

In the United States the battle against smoking has reached a peak. Doctors and health organizations are offering people many forms of help in their quest to quit this bad habit. In some of the chapters in this book I have gone into detail about ways to quit smoking, and which of them I consider worth trying.

The findings of a study by the U.S. Centers for Disease Control conducted between 1978 and 1994 revealed that 424,000 people die annually in the U.S. as a result of smoking. The yearly total cost (of medical and other expenditures) was an unbelievable $97 billion. It's no wonder that the tobacco industry has been sentenced to such high compensation payments.

If you stop smoking, you put on weight. So what?

The "change history method" can be a good way of quitting smoking. Even if by no longer smoking you were to "exchange" one problem with another – weight gain – you should not be discouraged.

I have an acquaintance who quit smoking 18 years ago, and did so overnight – this after he had tried to quit on at least three dozen occasions, and had smoked an average of 60 cigarettes a day.

I think he was able to quit with a kind of "change history method." After countless failures, the film in his mind all of a sudden "fitted." Sadly, this success also brought a disadvantage along with it. The man, who before had weighed around the average for his height and build, found that food tasted much better than before. He has gained about 2 pounds a year since he quit smoking. These excess pounds are certainly a risk factor for heart ailments (even though his blood readings are excellent), but I am quite certain that had he continued to smoke 60 cigarettes a day he would not have lived this long.

Interestingly, American doctors have a rule of thumb for such cases. A person who quits smoking should not waste any thought on his or her weight. On average people who quit smoking gain between 10 and 18 pounds. But smoking is more dangerous than being overweight.

You should accept a short-term weight gain. Don't try to quit smoking and to diet at the same time. Failure on both counts would be the inevitable result. Your brain can take a lot, but don't overtax it. You are careful about the way you treat your computer, aren't you?

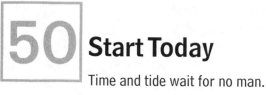

50 Start Today

Time and tide wait for no man.
Don't delay, begin today.

I have told you about my second wife, Barbara, and how easily she stopped smoking. She simply put her cigarettes away; no withdrawal treatment, no hypnosis, no nicotine chewing gum. She had a cold and didn't feel well. Cigarettes did not seem to taste good, so she stopped using them. Just like that.

> *Why all New Year's resolutions fail.*

I think that is the right way to go about it. If you want to change something in your life, why delay? Many people try to stop smoking or to start a diet on their birthday, on Christmas day, or on the 1st of January. A few days later they can again be seen puffing away or looking for tasty morsels in the refrigerator. Why? Because they were too ambitious. If you decide in December, for example, to stop smoking at the end of the year, you then begin a countdown. Two weeks to go ... one day ... another two hours ... five more minutes. On the stroke of midnight you extinguish your last cigarette and wait for the big moment. But nothing happens. You don't feel any better, so you start the next countdown. Now you ask yourself: how long will I be able to hold out?

After a week you are very satisfied with yourself. Admittedly you had a major argument with your partner in the meantime, your in-laws no longer talk to you, and your children have never been keener to spend the night with their grandmother. But you feel like a hero. A whole week without a single cigarette. That calls for a reward.

What would you like most? – A cigarette. Only one, of course. Then that's it. One cigarette won't harm anything. Just five minutes out of what has already been a week. Don't be fooled. With your first drag you are back where you started.

My suggestion is to start immediately if you want to change a habit. It doesn't matter if you succeed straight away. It's all right to try a few times before you get it right.

The cerebellum, the command headquarters of the brain for our habits, is constantly bombarded with new wishes until it finally absorbs them. Dr. Michael Gilewski of the famous Cedars Sinai Hospital in Los Angeles calls the cerebellum "our little friend that is always listening attentively." Habits are formed by nerve connections from the cerebellum to other parts of the brain. According to Dr. Gilewski, the more connections that are made, the stronger our habits are.

What I particularly like is that Gilewski – an enthusiastic marathon runner, by the way – is also fond of the rule "Start today!" This is the first step of a seven-step training program he has devised, which runs in full like this:

Step 1 Start today!
Don't delay. Get your doctor's OK and then begin.
Step 2 Just begin.
Don't start with a three-hour run. Grab a bike or walk around the block a few times. That's enough to start with.
Step 3 Be a winner.
Set a goal for yourself, one you can reach. Start with 20 minutes of walking, then increase this slowly. Take enough time off for sport, then you won't be under any pressure.
Step 4 Become an expert.
If you decide to start a sport, you should find out all about it. Treat it like you would a person you're attracted to. You want to get to know everything there is to know about them.

Step 5   Reward yourself.
Don't be too hard on yourself. When you have reached a reasonable goal you have set yourself, give yourself a day off.

Step 6   Be resilient.
A bad mood or bad weather should not keep you from your physical activity. There is only one good reason not to do it – when you're sick or injured.

Step 7   Find companions.
Nothing is more boring than running all alone for hours along a straight road. Find friends who are prepared to share your enthusiasm.

Nutrition, stress, environment, activity, attitude. In the five parts of this book I have tried to offer up my ideas on how to prevent heart disease. My last tip: whatever it is you want to do – eat better, stop smoking, reduce stress, think more positively – do it NOW. Your heart will thank you for it.

Epilogue

About 33 years ago now I became the first doctor to transplant a human heart. At that time, December 3, 1967, it was a medical sensation. Today it has almost become hospital routine. Medicine has made unbelievable progress since then. We hear almost daily of new developments that can improve our lives and even prolong them. But for many years medical research concentrated more on the "repair" of the patient than on the prevention of illness. That is the reason why I decided to write this book. I hoped to advise you, and to show you what you yourself can do to prevent heart trouble. You will have seen that there is a lot that you can do.

Many people have helped me to write the various chapters and I thank them all. Many who gave me encouragement or ideas are mentioned in this book, together with their findings.

My special thanks go to the staff of the library of the University of Cape Town for their assistance.

Vienna, Cape Town
December 2000

Heart of the World

Professor Christiaan Barnard's new foundation wants to help children and mothers in the world's poorest countries.

You all know Professor Christiaan Barnard, the famous heart specialist who was the first to transplant a human heart. What many people don't know is that Professor Barnard takes other people's welfare to heart in many ways. When he still worked at Cape Town's Groote Schuur hospital, he regularly operated on children from poor families free of charge. In this way he made a better future possible for many people and their families. With his Professor Christiaan Barnard Foundation he has now created an institution which wants to make a contribution towards a more humane 21st century.

The Foundation intends to help to improve the living conditions of the "heart of the world," its children, and mothers, particularly in poorer countries.

The Foundation intends to serve in three areas:

1 Addressing the population explosion
   The main focus is on Africa. The Foundation wants to support private theater groups and radio programs which try to put across the message of birth control.

2 Improving preventive health care
Geographical emphasis for the year 2000 is on Tibet and
Mozambique. The projects aim at the creation of primary health
care facilities including mother–child care centers.

3 Children in need
The Foundation intends to react to actual emergencies and to
help individual needy children. A project for the psychological
treatment of traumatized children from Kosovo, and the
treatment of girls and boys suffering from heart disease are
planned.

The Professor Christiaan Barnard Foundation is working in collab-
oration with several internationally renowned organizations. It
supports projects undertaken by local organizations and committed
private individuals.

References

American Heart Association. *Tools for a Better Lifestyle.* 1999

Barnard, C. *Das zweite Leben.* Munich 1993

Bell, D. *et al. Nie mehr müde, nie mehr schlapp.* Munich 1999

Biesalski, H. *Vitamine.* Stuttgart 1996

—. 'Antioxidative Vitamine in der Prävention'. *Deutsches Ärzteblatt Heft* 18/1995

—. *The Role of Antioxidative Vitamins in Primary and Secondary Prevention of Coronary Heart Disease.* Stuttgart 1999

Bloomfield, H. *Gegen jede Angst ist ein Kraut gewachsen.* Munich 1999

Byers, J. 'Effect of a Music Intervention on Noise Annoyance, Heart Rate, and Blood Pressure in Cardiac Surgery Patients'. *American Journal of Critical Care* 1997

Carper, J. *Jungbrunnen Nahrung.* Düsseldorf 1996

Collins, F. *Viagra. Das Ende der Impotenz.* Bern 1998

Elduff, P. 'How Much Alcohol and How Often?' *BMJ* 1997

Ernst, H. 'Reisen, um sich zu verändern'. *Psychologie heute* Nr. 7/1999

Fontana, D. *Mit dem Streß leben.* Bern 1991

Friend, T. 'Eggs May Not Hurt Cholesterol Level'. *USA Today* 1999

Gale, C. 'Vitamin C and Risk of Death From Stroke and Coronary Heart Disease in Cohort of Elderly People'. *BMJ* 1992

Gasser, R. *Die Kreta-Diät*. Niedernhausen/Ts 1998

Gerbert, F. 'Psychofalle Urlaub'. *Focus* 28/1999

Gerra, G. 'Neuroendocrine Responses of Health Volunteers to Techno-Music'. *International Journal of Psychophysiologie* 1998

Ghatak, A. 'Protective Role of Vitamin E and other Antioxidants in Heart Disease'. *Complementary Medicine* vol. 4/1998

Grobler, C. 'Stress in the workplace'. *CME* vol. 16/1998

Groman, E. *et al.* 'A Harmful Aid to Stopping Smoking'. *Lancet* vol. 353/ 1999

Gronbaek, M. 'Mortality Associated with Moderate Intake of Wine, Beer or Spirits'. *BMJ* 1998

Guzzetta, C. *Effects of Relaxation and Music Therapy on Patients in a Coronary Care Unit With Presumptive Acute Myocardial Infarction.* 1989

Hamm, M. *Das große Buch der Diäten*. Hamburg 1995

Hart, C. 'Alcohol Consumption and Mortality from All Causes, Coronary Heart Disease and Stroke'. *BMJ* 1999

Helberg, D. *Die Fit-For-Fun-Diät*. Hamburg 1995

Hembd, C. *Vitalstofftabelle*. Munich 1999

Holtmeier, H. *et al. Magnesium und Calcium*. Munich 1995

Hörzu Spezial Analyse von Grundnahrungsmitteln in einer Kaufhalle im Herbst 1996.

Huppertz, R. *et al. Hanfsamen und Hanföl*. Cologne 1997

Johnen, W. *Muskelentspannung nach Jacobson*. Munich 1995

Jones, F. *Mit Rotwein gegen Herzinfarkt*. Cologne 1996

Kempner, U. *Entspannung in der Mittagspause*. Niedernhausen/Ts 1998

Klepziq, H. *et al. Das kranke Herz*. Stuttgart 1993

Kluqe, H. *Heilkräuter. Die sanfte Hilfe der Natur*. Munich 1995

Knekt, P. *et al.* 'Flavonoid Intake and Coronary Mortality in Finland'. *BMJ* 1996

Kraaz, I. *Farbtherapie in der Küche*. Munich 1996

Kunze, U. *et al. Alternative Nicotine Delivery Systems (ANDS) — Public Health Aspects*. Vienna 1998

Law, M. 'Why Heart Disease Mortality is Low in France: The Time Lag Explanation'. *BMJ* 1999

Leendertse, J. 'Einfache Übung'. *Wirtschaftswoche* Nr. 30/1999

Leibold, G. *So werde ich Nichtraucher*. Augsburg 1998

Lemonick, M. 'Eat Your Heart Out'. *Time* vol. 154/1999

Lindemann, H. *Überleben im Streß*. Munich 1974

McLean, R. M. 'Magnesium and its Therapeutic Uses: A Review'. *American Journal of Medicine* 1994

Meryn, S. *et al. Der Mann 2000*. Vienna 1999

Möckel, T. *et al. Streßreduktion durch Musikhören*. Stuttgart 1995

Nager, F. *The Mythology of the Heart*. Basel 1993

Novotny, U. *Fit durch Fasten*. Munich 1999

Ornish, D. *Herzgesunde Kost*. Cologne 1998

Pollmer, U. *et al. Prost Mahlzeit!* Cologne 1994

—. *et al. Wohl bekomm's*. Cologne 1998

Prokop, L. *Lebenselexier Wein*. Graz 1995

Rath, M. *Nie wieder Herzinfarkt*. Munich 1996

Redtenbacher, H. *et al. Streß*. Leoben 1996

Schleicher, P. *Die sensationelle Kreta-Diät*. Munich 1999

Schlieper, C. A. *Grundfragen der Ernährung*. Hamburg 1992

Schlierf, D. *et al. Der Cholesterin-Ratgeber*. Stuttgart 1976

Schoberberqer, R. *et al. Nikotinabhängigkeit: Diagnostik und Therapie*. Vienna 1999

Scholz, H. *Mineralstoffe und Spurenelemente*. Stuttgart 1996

Schwarz, A. *et al. Gewürzheilkunde: Landsberg am Lech*. 1996

Singer, P. *Fisch gegen Herzinfarkt*. Frankfurt 1997

Singh, R. B. 'Magnesium Status and Risk of Coronary Artery Disease in Rural and Urban Population With Variable Magnesium Consumption'. *Magnes Res* 1997

Stampfer, M. J. *et al.* 'Vitamin E Consumption and the Risk of Coronary Disease in Women'. *New England Journal of Medicine* 1993

Stensvold, I. 'Cohort Study of Coffee Intake and Death from Coronary Heart Disease Over 12 Years'. *BMJ* 1996

Stephens, N. G. *et al.* 'Randomised Controlled Trial of Vitamin E in Patients With Coronary Disease: Cambridge Heart Antioxidant Study'. *Lancet* 1996

Tang, L. 'Mortality in Relation to Tar Yield of Cigarettes'. *BMJ* 1998

Tesar, E. *Mütter brauchen Zeit*. Vienna 1999

Treben, M. *Herz- & Kreislaufkrankheiten*. Steyr 1995

Weise, D. *Harmonische Ernährung*. Munich 1992

White, M. *Music Therapy: An Intervention to Reduce Anxiety in the Myocardial Infarction Patient.* 1992

Wollrinq, U. *Gymnastik im Herz- und Alterssport.* Aachen 1997

Yanker, G. *Walking.* Munich 1994

Index